Women's Sexual and Reproductive Health

Published by
Mzuni Press
P/Bag 201
Luwinga, Mzuzu 2

ISBN   978-99960-45-05-9
eISBN 978-99960-45-19-6

Mzuni Books no. 25

Mzuni Press is represented outside Africa by:
African Books Collective Oxford (orders@africanbookscollective.com)

www.mzunipress.blogspot.com
www.africanbookscollective.com

Printed with the assistance of the Deutsche Gesellschaft für Missions-wissenschaft

Women's Sexual and Reproductive Health, HIV/AIDS and the Anglican Church in Southern Malawi

Chimwemwe Kalalo

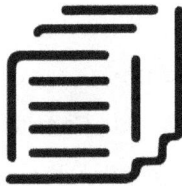

Mzuni Press

Mzuni Books no. 25

Mzuzu

2020

Abbreviations

AIDS	Acquired Immune Deficiency Syndrome
ARVs	Antiretroviral drugs
CLAIM	Christian Literature Association in Malawi
CPCA	Church of the Province of Central Africa (Malawi, Zambia, Zimbabwe and Botswana)
HIV	Human Immunodeficiency Virus
MANASO	Malawi Networks of Aids Service Organizations
MU	Mothers Union
NAC	National Aids Commission
PLWA	Person Living with Aids
PLWHIV	Person Living with HIV
TB	Tuberculosis Bacillus
UMCA	Universities Mission to Central Africa
UNAIDS	United Nations Joint Programme on HIV/AIDS.
VCT	Voluntary Counselling and Testing
WHO	World Health Organization
USGP	United Society for the Propagation of the Gospel

Contents

Introduction   7

Chapter 1:
The Anglican Church and St Luke's Hospital   11

Chapter 2:
Women's Experiences in Sexual and Reproductive Health   17

Chapter 3:
The Anglican Church and Women's Sexuality   77

Chapter 4:
Faith versus Reality: A Diet that is not Balanced   115

Bibliography   120

Appendices   127

Index   137

Introduction

Although research shows that a great percentage of the Malawian population is quite knowledgeable about HIV/Aids transmission and prevention, the epidemic still continues to kill at a fast rate, and the government and other stakeholders including the faith communities are continuously meeting the challenges of HIV/Aids.

As everyone fights Aids, one important area to consider in curbing the virus and improving support for infected people is the satisfaction of a woman's reproductive and sexual needs. The coming of the Aids epidemic has greatly influenced a woman's sexual and reproductive health. As it is the responsibility of every individual to meet the challenges of HIV/Aids, proper management of her sexual and reproductive life would consequently have a potential benefit to the whole family and the nation at large. Improving her health means improving the health of her partner and her children as well. Sexual and reproductive health is a key component of health and quality of life.

Women's sexual reproductive health is a challenge today because sexuality is explicitly related to HIV/Aids, a disease that has no cure.[1] How a woman handles her sexual and reproductive life is very crucial today. When a woman's health is poor sexually, it gives room for HIV entry. This can ruin not only her health but also other lives as well including the infants born to her. Many women in Malawi have died, infected and affected by the HIV pandemic because of, among other factors, a negative approach to their own sexuality. Women could be able to improve their reproductive health if they are knowledgeable about and in control of their sexuality and sexual relations. Culture, economy, ethics and values do influence a woman's sexual health, consequently affecting the whole family. By coming up with responsible sexual and reproductive choices such as, safe and healthy pregnancy,

---

[1]   See Overton Mzunda et al, *The God of Love and Compassion: A Christian Meditation on Aids*, Zomba: Kachere, 2002. The authors cite the understanding of sexuality as one of the problems in addressing the AIDS pandemic, p. 5.

family planning, safe delivery, sexuality education, when to have sex and with whom, HIV/Aids could be defeated.

The National Aids Control Programme shows a high HIV prevalence rate of women attending antenatal clinics. The rate varies from 10% in the rural areas to 35% in urban areas. In 2001, out of 7361 pregnant women sampled at Queen Elizabeth Central Hospital, 20% tested positive.[2] This high infection rate suggests that many children are born HIV positive. There is again evidence that HIV infection in women of the reproductive age group is between 4 to 6 times higher than with their male counterparts. In 2003, out of 760,000 infected adults, 58% were women with 45,000 newly infected ones as compared to 35,000 among men.[3]

In the mid 19th century when Christianity was introduced into Malawi, the missionaries took great concern at improving people's health. One such mission was the Universities Mission to Central Africa as a pioneer of the Anglican Church in Malawi. Since then to the present, the Church has worked as a team with the government in the provision of medical services in Malawi and in its fight against HIV/Aids

This book therefore looks at how adequately the Anglican Church in the Upper Shire Diocese responds to the issue of women's sexual reproductive health in the context of HIV/Aids. It is anticipated that this work will serve as a valuable tool for pastoral care not only to members of the faith community but even to all persons who are still uncertain on how to handle women's sexual reproductive issues.

Child bearing exposes women to many health risks. Complications from pregnancy and childbirth are a major cause of women's deaths in Malawi. Transmission rates of STDs (including HIV) are higher in women and if not treated and prevented have many complications such as infertility, genital cancer, ectopic pregnancy and even death. Thus,

---

[2] "HIV/Syphilis Sero Prevalence in Antenatal Clinic Attendees: NAC Malawi Sentinel Surveillance Report 2001", p. 8.

[3] National Aids Commission, *HIV/Aids in Malawi: 2003 Estimates and Implications*, Lilongwe: January 2004.

ignoring contraceptive and pregnancy related issues could seriously affect the women's health and may lead to prenatal HIV transmission.

The use of condoms as a device for preventing the transmission of HIV and other STDs is and has been an issue of hot debate among the faith communities since most churches value abstinence and faithfulness in marriage as the only way of curbing the virus. In many faith communities, a condom is still a taboo and still being viewed as a tool of promiscuity. There is again a culture of silence in most churches on women's sexual and reproductive health. Culturally too most men refuse to use a condom that could offer some protection to the wife from contracting any sexually transmitted infection. The faith community has therefore an important role to play in enhancing the position of women and changing accepted norms. Improving the status of women is not only a matter of theology but of ethics, health and survival. This challenges churches to change some of their attitudes and visions and to undertake new and creative initiatives in their pastoral ministry. A crisis such as Aids should be a time of opportunity and of decision-making.[4]

I conducted this research project not merely as a theologian but more especially as a woman, a widow, and one who has not only been affected by the HIV/Aids epidemic but infected too, living with the virus. The loss of my husband, my only child (the child I never saw) and later my being diagnosed HIV positive came as a nightmare and a tragedy into my life. It has given me a whole new outlook on the suffering that Aids brings into a family. The bitterer I became about my situation, the more I was forced to do something. It was this experience that forced me to contribute to and write on improving a woman's sexual reproductive health. Being part of the "group", I am concerned about the Aids situation in Malawi. The challenges of widowhood, the pain, shame and humiliation that go with the disease are things that pierce my heart. Yet it makes me proud to write this thesis from an inside experience.

---

[4] Gillian Patterson, *Love in Time of Aids: Women Health and the Challenge of HIV/Aids*, Geneva: WCC, 1996, p. 1.

Chapter 1: The Anglican Church and St Luke's Hospital

Christianity in Malawi traces its history back over one hundred and fifty years to the first mission. Under the influence of David Livingstone, explorer and missionary from Scotland, mission groups reached Malawi hoping to open up Africa by bringing Christianity and abolishing the slave trade.[1]

The University Mission to Central Africa, popularly known as UMCA, was the first of the pioneer missions to land in Malawi in the 19th Century. It was this classical mission that pioneered the present-day Anglican Church in Malawi.

Following his extensive journeys in central Africa, Livingstone went back to England in December 1856, alarmed by the slave trade. In his address at Cambridge University he reported the appalling conditions of people in Central Africa and begged his audiences in Britain to draw their attention there and plant a mission in Central Africa. His plea was, "I go back to Africa to try to make an open path for commerce and Christianity. Do you carry out the work, which I have begun, I leave it with you!"[2]

---

[1] David Livingstone was born on 19th March 1813 at Blantyre in Scotland. After completing his education at Glasgow University where he was trained as a medical doctor, Livingstone was convinced that he was called to be a missionary. He desired to explore the continent of Africa which was referred to by many Europeans as the "Dark Continent." In December 1840, he left England for Africa and reached Malawi in September 1859. During his missionary journeys, Livingstone was certain that missions were essential in Central Africa. His last journey saw his death at Chitambo village in northern Zambia on 1 May 1873. For more details about his life see Jack Simmons, *Livingstone and Africa*, London: English Universities Press, 1955.

[2] A.E.M. Anderson-Morshead, *The History of the Universities Mission to Central Africa 1859-1909*, London: UMCA, 1953, vol. 1, p. 3. This famous lecture took place at the Senate House in Cambridge on 4th December 1857. See also, George Shepperson, "Livingstone and the Years of Preparation 1813-1857" in

The first UMCA group comprising 14 lay and clerical missionaries sailed for Africa in October 1860. The group included Fredrick Mackenzie, who was to be consecrated bishop in Cape Town, Rev Lovell Procter, Rev Henry Scudamore, Horace Waller, Samuel Gamble and Alfred Adams.[3] Their purpose was to found an agricultural village that should show the natives how to produce cotton for export; show them the truths of the Christian religion, and display in its corporate life the model of a Christian and civilized community; and thus, by their presence, their example and their economy, they would begin to destroy slavery.[4] The missionaries landed in Malawi in 1861 under the leadership of Bishop Fredrick Mackenzie, a man who won people's confidence and trust.[5] According to Jonathan Newell,

> His fine manly form and presence not only indicated his great physical capacity for such a work, but caused everyone who saw him to think instinctively of the homage which savage natives ever pay to personal endowments and physical powers such as his and the great advantage that they would thus gain in dealing with him.[6]

With David Livingstone leading the way, the group reached Chibisa village in Chikwawa district about 200 km up the Shire in the area of chief Mankhokwe. Within a short time, they moved further north and

---

Bridglal Pachai (ed), *Livingstone. Man of Africa: Memorial Essays 1873-1973*, London: Longman, 1973.

[3] Philip Elston, "Livingstone and the Anglican Church", in Bridglal Pachai, *Livingstone. Man of Africa: Memorial Essays*, p. 73. Rev Henry Scudamore died on February 22, 1862. His tomb still stands at Magomero.

[4] J.M. Schoffeleers, "Livingstone and the Mang'anja Chiefs", in Bridglal Pachai, *Livingstone. Man of Africa: Memorial Essays 1873-1973*, p. 123.

[5] Phillip Elston, "Livingstone and the Anglican Church", in Bridglal Pachai, *Livingstone, Man of Africa*, p. 73. Fredrick Mackenzie was the Archdeacon of Natal in South Africa. He was consecrated the first Anglican missionary bishop of the people of Nyasa and the Shire River on 1st January 1861 at St George's Cathedral, Cape Town, by Bishop Gray.

[6] Jonathan Newell, "Not War but Defence of the Oppressed? Bishop Mackenzie's Skirmishes with the Yao in 1861", in Kenneth R. Ross (ed), *Faith at the Frontiers of Knowledge*, Blantyre: CLAIM-Kachere, 1998, p. 130.

settled at Magomero in Chiradzulu district in the Shire Highlands among the Mang'anja people. Being on a slave-trading route, the site offered the missionaries an opportunity to fight the human trade easily and to block the passage, thus, offering a quasi-military refuge for local people. The Namadzi River was advantageous to the missionaries who could build a stockade for protection.[7]

Zanzibar offered easy communications to Europe and a stable government offered them freedom to carry out their work and at the same time diminished their fear of being attacked by hostile tribes. By 1868, arrangements were being sought to bring the mission back to Malawi.[8] It was only in 1881 when the mission finally landed on Malawi soil for the second time. Led by Rev William Percival Johnson and Chauncy Maples, the group settled at Chitesi village on the eastern side of Lake Malawi. The intention of the two priests was to evangelize not only the eastern side of the Lake but to go further to the western side. In 1885, they moved to Likoma Island which then became the headquarters of the mission.[9] It was mandated to oversee all outstations.

The end of the 19th century saw many African states being taken over by the European squads. Historians term this the "scramble for Africa." Others call it the partition of Africa. Here in Malawi, the partition affected the UMCA mission at Likoma, as most of its mission stations along the eastern side of the lake fell to the Portuguese who were at

---

[7] G.H. Wilson, *The History of the Universities Mission to Central Africa*, London: UMCA, 1955, p. 11.

[8] The key figures that played a big role in the mission's move to Malawi were Chauncy Maples and William Johnson. Maples was in charge of the mission until 1895. On the life of Maples, see E. Maples, *Chauncy Maples: Pioneer Missionary in East and Central Africa for Nineteen Years and Bishop of Likoma, Lake Nyasa*, London: Longman, 1897. Rev. W.P. Johnson was an archdeacon from 1876 to 1928. For his biography see Beryl Brough, An Evaluation of the Work of Archdeacon William Percival Johnson in Nyasaland (1876-1928), MTh, University of Glamorgan, 1997.

[9] The word "likoma" means "beautiful and without any defects." The early inhabitants of the place found the area endowed with beauty and named it "chalo chokoma."

the same time Catholics.[10] It was this situation that led the mission to concentrate also on the west of the lake. Their first target was Nkhotakota, 100 km away. Despite forces they met in the area that could have hindered their stay, the mission succeeded in establishing a station at Nkhotakota in 1894.[11] Rev. Arthur Sim was in charge of the mission up to 1895 when J. Wimbush took over. Within a short time, schools were opened. The UMCA did not concentrate their work only in Likoma and Nkhotakota. In the Shire area, they reached Malindi, Matope and Likwenu.[12] Today these parishes are part of the Upper Shire Diocese.

One of the lessons learnt during its first years was to involve the Africans actively in the missionary work. The missionaries tried to develop an indigenous ministry with African features.[13] The period saw frequent baptisms and ordinations of many Africans to the post of deacons and even higher positions. Even in their educational systems they relied heavily on African teachers, especially those they had brought from Zanzibar. Such people included Augustine Ambali, Yohana Abdallah, Michael Hamisi and Leonard Kamungu.[14] From Malawi, the UMCA expanded further into Zambia at a place called Morose, a mission in the

---

[10] *Central African History for the Malawi School Certificate of Education*, Lilongwe: Ministry of Education and Culture, 1992, p. 105.

[11] Ibid. At Nkhotakota they met not only the British control but also the Muslim influence and the Scottish missionaries who wanted to open their own station there. However, Harry Johnston favoured the UMCA against the Scottish missions.

[12] Phillip Elston, "A Note on the Universities Mission to Central Africa: 1859-1914," p. 360. Likwenu became an important station by 1914.

[13] James Tengatenga, *Church, State and Society in Malawi: The Anglican Case*, Zomba: Kachere, 2006.

[14] For the autobiographies of Ambali and Abdallah, see Augustine Ambali, "Thirty Years in Nyasaland," London: UMCA, 1931 and Yohana Abdallah, "The Yaos: Chiikala cha Wayao," Zomba: Government Press, 1919.

care of Leonard Kamungu, who became the first Nyanja priest in 1902.[15] This African ministry made great progress under Bishop Trower.[16]

Dioceses in the Anglican Church in Malawi

The Anglican Church of Malawi as one of the mainline churches has about 300,000 members (2005). The first Malawian to become a bishop of the Anglican Church was Josiah Mtekateka.[17] In the 20th Century, the diocese of Nyasaland witnessed a demarcation that resulted in four dioceses for easy management. The diocese of Lake Malawi was established in 1951 and consisted of areas in the northern and central regions of Malawi.[18] Southern Malawi Diocese was opened in 1971. Its first Bishop was Donald Arden who resigned in 1976. The Northern Malawi Diocese was established on 1st January 1995. The dioceses of Upper Shire and Southern Malawi comprise all districts in southern Malawi including part of Ntcheu in the central region.[19]

---

[15] Leonard Kamungu was among the first pupils when Chia School was opened in 1887. He was a Malawian missionary who served in Malawi and Zambia. He died in 1913. Kamungu is commemorated annually on 27th February for his missionary work. For more details on Kamungu, see John Weller, *The Priest from the Lakeside: the Story of Leonard Kamungu of Malawi and Zambia 1877-1913*, Blantyre: CLAIM, 1971.

[16] See Bridglal Pachai, *Livingstone Man of Africa: Memorial Essays 1873-1973*, London: Longman, 1973.

[17] He was consecrated in St Peter's Cathedral on May 27, 1965. For details about his life, see Denis M'passou, *Josiah Mtekateka: From a Priest's Dog-Boy to a Bishop*, Chilema, 1979. Habil Matthew Chipembere was ordained an Anglican priest on 21.1.1938. He was twice considered to become the Anglican Church's first black bishop in Malawi, but was dropped both times for being the father of a radical son, Masauko. See Masauko Chipembere, *Hero of the Nation*, ed. by Robert Rotberg, Blantyre: CLAIM-Kachere, 2000, p. 183.

[18] "Constitution and Canons: Church of the Province of Central Africa", 1996, p. 17. This excludes part of Ntcheu district to the southeast and western part of Lake Malawi i.e. to the Peak of Chilobwe Mountain between Lizulu and Mlangeni and part of Golomoti.

[19] Ibid.

The Catchment Area of the Upper Shire Diocese

The Upper Shire diocese stretches from Mangochi to Namadzi River and consists of five components called archdeaconries. They are under the leadership of archdeacons who are the senior priests. Zomba archdeaconry consists of Zomba, Likwenu, Chinamwali, Magomero and the sub parish of Jali; Balaka archdeaconry comprises Liwonde, Balaka, Namalomba and Ntcheu parishes. Under Mangochi West archdeaconry are Mangochi, Mpinganjira, Mpondasi, Mchenga, Mkope, Monkey Bay and Katema parishes. Mangochi East contains Malindi, Makanjira (Lungwena), Chingwenya (Namwera), and Masuku parishes. Finally, Shire archdeaconry caters for Lisungwi (Phalula), Matope, Chilipa, Chinseu and Mwanza parishes. The diocese has about 46,000 members.[20]

The Medical Department—St Luke's Hospital

The division of the Southern Malawi diocese not only involved parishes but also the institutions. St Luke's Hospital is one of the institutions Upper Shire Diocese benefited from the division. Malindi hospital and eight health centers in Machinga, Mwanza, Zomba and Mangochi districts also form part of the medical department. These health centers are Mkope, Mpondasi, Lulanga, Nkasala, Matope, Chilipa, Mposa and Gawanani.

---

[20] Int. Francis Chipala, Likwenu parish priest, Chilema, 8.9.04. This is just a rough estimation. Chipala confessed that it is not possible to come up with statistical figures of the whole diocese as of now. Hopefully in the near future.

Chapter 2: Women's Experiences in Sexual and Reproductive Health

Women's sexual and reproductive health is a big challenge to the church, especially today in the time of HIV/Aids. How the church approaches the subject has some impact on the life of a woman as a whole. The book deals with the Anglican Church and how it has involved itself in its pastoral ministry to include women's sexual and reproductive issues in today's context of HIV/Aids. This is mainly discussed in the next chapter. This chapter therefore explores and depicts the experiences and real challenges women go through concerning their sexual and reproductive health.

To write women's experiences from a woman's perspective is to satisfy the desires of many modern historians who realize that most histories in the past have been written from a male perspective.[25]

I was glad indeed to see that the women had confidence in me. They opened up and confided in me as a fellow woman. My own part as a widow, my HIV positive status, my being an ARV client played a major role in the study. I was open to disclose myself as a widow to other widows and we could share challenges of widowhood. I would also declare my HIV status where appropriate. This as well motivated many women. And I believe that although most women still fear to know their HIV status, my own story has given some of them some hope. Talking to ARV clients was again easy because we know each other as we meet every month at the same hospital to get the drugs. Here, we shared experiences and challenges as well.

Birth Experiences

While birth marks the creation of life, it is for most women the most severe physical ordeal they will ever experience. Most women stated that giving birth was a nasty experience and they just did it because it is nature. For a child to be born, it takes a long way. A journey that is not

---

[25] See Rachel Banda, *Women of Bible and Culture,* Zomba: Kachere, 2005, p. 15. .

17

only challenging and traumatic but which also leads to joy at the sight of the newborn baby. Consequently, this experience may affect the reproductive health of the mother.

Pregnancy

After conception, the woman has the responsibility of taking care of the foetus in her womb for 9 months. To most women, this is not an easy period. Care for pregnancy is challenging and requires adequate support from the husband, the family and the community at large. Women from Malemia described the challenges they faced during pregnancy. Pregnancy experiences are unique to every woman but most face similar challenges. Many physical changes take place in her body during pregnancy. During pregnancy, many women lose appetite, vomit and have backaches, fever, swollen breasts, painful waist and stomach aches. These illnesses are normal and occur to most pregnant women. A few women experienced pain below their navel and had problems with high blood pressure that usually resulted in swollen legs and feet. It is again usual for most women to feel nausea, crave for certain foods and at the same time resent some, such as meat, eggs and rice when they are pregnant.[26] Some do not even want to be close to their partners during such periods.

> I loathe having sex with him because to me he has a very bad odour, especially in his mouth, even with thorough washing.[27]

This is the period when partners need not only to be supportive but also to understand some of these novel attitudes, otherwise it is very easy to be irritated and lose one's temper. Haemorrhoids also seem to be

---

[26] This usually happens in the first trimester of the pregnancy, i.e. the first 13 weeks.

[27] Int. Woman 16, 11.1.2005. *Amandinyansa kuti agone nane. Amanunkha ndi mkamwa momwe olo atsuke chotani*. He despises me when he wants to sleep with me. He smells including the mouth despite thorough washing.

common to most pregnant women.[28] It is, however, strange that even after delivery, this nasty illness continues to hurt many of them.

A pregnant mother should not look gloomy but cheerful. The baby inside does likewise, it is gloomy. This is why some women bear fragile and weak babies. You cannot hide a pregnancy. It will still come out on its own. So, the best thing is always to be in good spirits, caressing it at times, that the baby inside should be feeling jovial.[29]

When pregnant, every woman wants the birth of her baby to be a positive experience. As such, she expects every help, advice and support to make the most of her experience. Women from Malemia lamented that there is little advice and support given to pregnant women from their faith communities. This is perhaps done unintentionally, but most faith communities may not see the need to do so. At times, they may not even know what advice or support to give to such women.

> This is a crucial moment when you are anxious of what will come out of your belly. It is important to pray and seek favour from God that you should bear a live child and without defect.[30]

Counselling of pregnant women is mainly left in the hands of elderly women.[31] They advise on postures such as how to stretch one's legs when seated and not bending one's back when walking. A pregnant

---

[28] These are swollen enlarged veins that sit just inside or outside the opening of the anus. It leads to irritation of the skin and bleeding when opening bowels. Most women experience this in the second stage of their pregnancy between 14 to 26 weeks.

[29] Int. Woman 6, 5.5.2005. *Mzimayiwapakati asamakhumate, osati nkhwi-nyiliri koma kumasangalala. Naye wamkatiyo amachitanso chimodzimodzi kukhumatanso. Ndiye pobereka ndi aja ena amabereka khanda lofoka, lopanda mphamvu. Mimba siibisika. Ngakhale ubise imatuluka basi. Chofunika ndi kusangalala, ukakhala kumaisisita kuti mwana azimva kukomedwa mkati.*

[30] Int. Woman 23, 14.1.2005. *Iyi ndi nthawi yoopsa yofunika kupemphera. Sumadziwa kuti chidzatuluke ndi chiyani. Ndi bwino kumapemphera kuti Mulungu akutsogolere udzabeleke mwana wa moyo ndinso opanda chilema.*

[31] These are not necessarily "anankungwi" but any elderly women such as a mother, a granny or an aunt.

mother is also advised not to stand on the doorway otherwise the baby will do likewise. This would give her problems during delivery.[32] Standing on the door is like blocking the way for people to pass, including the baby inside.[33] A pregnant mother must not eat eggs. Even drinking water while standing is prohibited as the baby upon birth would vomit through the nose and this would be dangerous.[34] From my sample, most women said they adhere to such practices for their own good. Few women said they did not see any connection between delivering and adhering to such practices. They said they could agree with the tradition of good posture but not with the others.

> I cannot manage that. I will always be forgetting. I also do not see any connection between delivery and standing on the doorway. I have children whom I delivered without problems.[35]

Another *mwambo* given to a pregnant mother is to immediately untie the firewood sheaf upon arrival from the bush. Failure to do so will result in her tying herself and therefore having difficulties at delivery.[36] *Mwambo* is also given on decency in dress. A pregnant mother is to dress modestly.

> Dressing. A pregnant mother needs to be respected. Do not wear tight clothes. The skirt must be loose enough. She should not cover herself around her shoulders.[37]

---

[32] Compare with the traditions of Tumbuka people in Alister Munthali, Change and Continuity: Perceptions about Childhood Diseases among the Tumbuka of Northern Malawi, Rhodes University, 2002, p. 128.

[33] Int. Woman 10, 30.4.2005.

[34] Ibid.

[35] Int. Woman 41, 17.1.2005. *Sindingazikwanitse zimenezo. Ndingathe kumaiwala. Sindimawonaso kusiyana kulikonse pakati pa kubereka ndi kuyima pakhomo. Ndili ndi ana ndinaberekanso bwino bwino.*

[36] Int. Woman 10, 30.4.2005.

[37] Int. Woman 3, Malemia, 9.1.2005. *Kavalidwe. Mayi wapakati amafunika kudzilemekeza. Osavala chovala chothina, siketi izikhala ya chingwe kuti azitha kutakasuka. Osafunda nsalu mmapewa.*

The hospital staff plays a big role in counselling. This is mainly done at antenatal clinics. Most women start antenatal clinics when the pregnancy is 3 or 4 months old. Many women praised the good services they get from hospitals. Counselling during antenatal is supported by a number of songs such as the ones below.

Song 1:

One:
Mlera ine mulera. x2
Ana onsewa mulera,
Ndikhale olera ine mulera? x2

I care for the children. x2
All these children
Should I be the one to care for all these children?

All:
Mlera ine mulera x2
Ana onsewa mulera,
Ndikhale olera ine mulera? x2

I care for the children. x2
All these children
Should I be the one to care for all these children?

Song 2:
One: Kusikelo kulibe wolemera
Kusikelo kulibe wodya bwino
Kusikelo kulibe wophunzira

At Antenatal, no one is rich.
no one eats well
no one is educated. [It does not matter.]

All: Kusikelo kulibe wolemera. x2
One: Inde, tetee. x2
All: Eeeh
One: Tetetetetee
All: Kusikelo kulibe wolemera.

At Antenatal, no one is rich.
Yes, teteee.
Eeeh
Tetetetetee
At Antenatal no one is rich.

Quite a good number of women visit St Luke's Hospital. In 2004, 7797 women visited the antenatal clinics.[38] Most women commended the care and treatment they get but complained of inadequate drugs. Panadol seems to be the obvious medicine for every illness.

---

[38] The statistics was collected from the public health department at St Luke's from January to December, 2004. Antenatal clinic is done Monday to Friday from 8 am.

21

Some illnesses require a stronger drug. Some of us have problems with backache, unusual vomit and paining legs. But each time we come here, we get Panadol.[39]

Delivery Experience

Delivery time is the climax of the birthing experience. No woman can forget the actual pushing, the pressure and the feeling of a baby coming out. It is a weird experience. To most women, labour is spontaneous. About 90% of the women interviewed had their delivery at the hospital. Only 10% delivered with the help of traditional birth attendants. For many women, going to hospitals has the advantage of safe delivery.[40] Although most of them felt that traditional attendants were better in terms of how they care and treat patients unlike with hospital personnel most of whom are rough and harsh, they still prefer the hospital. To most women, traditional birth attendants do not have enough and reliable equipment, and they feel that today in the context of HIV/Aids, it is not safe to deliver at the traditional attendants.

Let me get the HIV virus from other places, not at a traditional birth attendant's who does not even possess gloves.[41]

A small percentage of women who prefer to deliver at home said that they do so because of the way some midwives behave in hospitals. One

---

[39] Int. Woman 44, 17.1.2005. The hospital staff admitted this lack of sufficient drugs at the hospital, which has indeed affected the hospital's operations.

[40] Compare Evelyn Chinguwo, "Safe Motherhood: Constraints to Women's Utilization of Maternal Services in Zomba and Nsanje Districts", July 1995, UNIMA, MA. Chinguwo's study reveals that most women fail to utilize maternal services because of the socio-economic and cultural framework in which they operate and make decisions. Her findings revealed that removing this framework would help influence more women to use hospital based maternal services. My findings however do not mean that this structure is no longer there. I believe it is a result of social change. Both men and women today see the need to go to the hospital for delivery. Perhaps it is indeed out of fear of HIV/Aids as some women suggested. Whatever the cause, this is a positive development.

[41] Int. Woman 32, 25.1.2005.

woman who had been disappointed with the hospital staff had this to say:

> I will never visit the hospital again for delivery. I still remember how I lost my baby in 2002 because of carelessness from the midwives on duty. I was in labour and kept calling for the nurse to come and help as I was feeling the baby coming out. The nurses took no notice of me and were busy drinking tea in their office. All they said was – "Siinakwane nthawi mmadziwa chiyani kodi inu? Mungotisokosa basi?" (It is not yet time. What do you know about delivery? You are just troubling us). It was already too late when they came, only to find the baby about to drop, but not breathing. I strongly believe this could not have happened had the nurse cared for me.[42]

This lady now has a one-year-old baby. She delivered at home with a traditional birth attendant. According to her, she was given the respect due to a pregnant mother and she does not regret visiting her. This lady believes that one can get HIV/Aids anywhere even in the hospitals where people claim that it is a safe place.

> I have three children all delivered at home by my own mother. I have never experienced any delivery problems as those experienced by most women in hospitals such as *kuchepa njira* (small cervical canal), or be delivered with forceps that usually leave bruises. I have never had a still birth either.[43]

On how they are received at the hospital, most women did not give high praise for the medical staff, as they felt that they were not accorded the respect they deserve at the maternity ward. They said that hospital personnel are harsh and rude.

> Some midwives behave as if they are not women and shout at us and talk in bad language. Sometimes, some midwives send *okolopa* (ward attendants) to attend to you when they are busy drinking tea. Many midwives are emotional, always screaming and shouting. *Mmene mumachitira ndi amuna anuwo mumayesa mwana adzatulukira komwera tiyi.* ('The time you were making love with

---

[42] Int. Woman 24, 14.1.2005.

[43] Int. Woman 27, 16.1.2005.

your man, you thought the baby will come out like the way you drink tea').[44]

This negative experience envelops most women. Although the standard of care differs from hospital to hospital depending on the midwife on duty, most women gave the same sentiments. Some women commented that some nurses leave mothers to give birth unattended.[45]

I delivered my child alone when I got tired of calling the nurse on duty to help me.[46]

Many women talk about negative delivery experiences. Caesarean sections are done far too often these days.[47] Most women interviewed who had more than three children talked of at least one Caesarean section experience.

I have four children, all of which I delivered through Caesarean section.[48]

Most women fear Caesarean deliveries. This, they said, is the last thing they would do.[49] Most of those who go through normal deliveries

---

[44] Int. Woman 19, 11.1.2005.

[45] The then Archbishop of the Anglican Central African Province, Bernard Malango, discouraged such behaviour. In his speech to graduating nurses at St Luke's College of Nursing in Malosa in April 2005, Malango noted that negligence in some medical practitioners in hospitals has greatly contributed to maternal and infant deaths (*The Nation,* 19.4.2005, p. 3). Malango added that this attitude has painted a bad picture of health service delivery in the country and needs to be changed. After his retirement , Bishop Malango was replaced by father Brighton Malasa, then, the Bishop's chaplain.

[46] Int. Woman 5, 9.1.2005. *Ine mwana wanga ndinabereka ndekha nditatopa ndikuitana adokotala.*

[47] HIV increases the number of Caesarian sections. Women that are HIV positive and pregnant are often advised to go for Caesar.

[48] Int. Woman 7, 10.1.2005.

[49] From my study, not even a single woman would choose Caesarean should it be optional. Those that had undergone Caesar did so not out of choice but emergency, after failing to give birth normally. Surprisingly, most women said even if they were HIV positive and pregnant, they could not opt for Caesar. I

complained of difficult deliveries. While some complained of a prolonged labour period, most women have problems with the size of their cervical canal. Many of these were delivered with forceps. Some women undergo induction.[50] Women who have undergone this say the pain is just unbearable.

> This was my third pregnancy. The other two were normal and did not give me much pain. But this one mmm *mavuto* (trouble). I stayed in the labour room for the whole day pushing and pushing. At last I was told induction was the only remedy. I did not even know what it was and of course I had no option. My cervix was closed so they had to use forceps. *Mwana amazunza* (child bearing is painful).[51]

Another woman commented on a bad experience she went through in 1983.

> I have six children. The first five did not give me much trouble as this last one. Labour took too long. My cervix was closed. In the end the midwife boiled some water to speed the coming of the baby. Unfortunately, the heat of the water burnt me, leaving me with bruises. I still have the scars today. This was a nasty experience. She is my last child.[52]

Still Birth Delivery

When going for delivery every woman has high expectations and looks forward to see the coming baby. It is a tragedy to every woman to lose a baby at birth. Stillbirth deliveries are common these days and it is a bad experience. In 2004, 64 still birth deliveries were recorded at St

---

went through Caesar myself and personally feel this is the best way of delivery. And should I have a second pregnancy, Caesarian section will be my choice.

[50] When labour is difficult, midwives use medical drugs to induce it.

[51] Int. Woman 29, 18.1.2005.

[52] Int. Woman 14, 10.1.2005. In the past, this system of boiling hot water was common. But today it is being discouraged for it is becoming more dangerous not only to the baby but to the mother as well.

Luke's Hospital. Though the percentage seems small, 64 deaths is quite a big number.

St Luke's delivery cases for January to December 2004

Total deliveries = 1397 births		
Normal births (SVDs)[53]	1298	88 %
C/S (Caesarean section)	92	6 %
Still birth	64	4 %
V/X (Vertex extraction)[54]	43	3 %

It is sad to bear the agony of a child dying. I can recall my own experience on 24th July 2002 when I lost my daughter I had looked forward to nurse. When I discovered I was pregnant, I shed tears of joy. I shed tears with labour pains. As I made my way to the theatre for a Caesarian section, I shed tears of expectation. The final painful tear was shed when I heard I had lost the baby. Everything was just too much. It was the first and worst Caesarean experience I will never forget.[55]

One woman commented about her birthing experience as follows

> It was in 2001 when I fell pregnant. I used to have high blood pressure. When I was nearing my days, I had convulsions right there in the ward. In the labour ward my blood pressure shot up again. I

---

[53] SVD is an abbreviation for Spontaneous Vertex Deliveries.

[54] This is also called forceps delivery using instruments.

[55] I was a month pre due, labour started spontaneously during the night of 23rd July. I was rushed to the hospital to see my doctor who knew beforehand that I was going for Caesar. Though I was already in labour, nurses did their job as usual, checking BP, cervical canal etc. This took time and by the time I was rushed to the theatre I was bleeding. The operation too took longer than I expected - about 5 hrs. This I was told by my aunt who said that she had already started crying outside the theatre room when the time was taking long. My daughter was alive but failed to gasp breath. She tried to inhale some oxygen but it failed. She died. What went wrong, only God knows. May be I was late; maybe I had infected her, maybe.

had convulsion too. After gaining my senses, the baby had stopped breathing, and was dead. I strongly believe my people at home bewitched me.[56]

Many things, such as the following, cause stillbirths and other delivery problems to mothers during their birthing experience.[57]

Kung'ambika chibelekero (broken uterus). One service provider commented that most women who start visiting traditional birth attendant realize too late that they have some complications, which can only be sorted out by medical personnel. By the time they reach the hospital, their uterus is already broken and most lose a lot of blood as a result. Some women even die from that.

Another problem is anemia because of lack of sufficient and appropriate food for pregnant women in their homes. This results in difficult delivery. Anemia is often associated with HIV/Aids.

Failure to have normal deliveries due to early pregnancies.

Those that are HIV positive and pregnant encounter many problems because of their low immune system. Most of them have Caesarean delivery because they are already weak.

Another service provider added that some women meet challenges during delivery because of old age. They lie about their age and the number of children they have.[58] A few women believe stillbirths, miscarriages and other delivery problems are a result of negligence with regard to sexual taboos.[59] According to them, most pregnant mothers

---

[56] Int. Woman 21, 12.1.2005.

[57] Int. F. Kachingwe, midwife, St Luke's hospital, 30.1.2005.

[58] Int. Mrs Maloya, nurse, St Luke's hospital, 19.1.2005. She commented that one way to improve women's sexual reproductive health is to increase health talk at community level and at the same time encourage partners to follow their spouses to the antenatal clinic.

[59] Int. Woman 10, 30.4.2005. This lady refuted any association of witchcraft or evil spirits to one's miscarriage or stillbirth. For comparative analysis, see Alister Munthali, Change and Continuity: Perceptions about Childhood Diseases among the Tumbuka of Northern Malawi, Rhodes University, 2002, p. 134. Writing about the birth rituals among the Tumbuka, Munthali reports that

today do not adhere to the counsel of the old on how to care for the pregnancy.

> In our days, we never encountered any problems like these you are having today. There was no vomiting and ill health because of pregnancy. Even at delivery, we never faced problems. Most mothers were delivering at their homes with traditional attendants. The reason was because we adhered to the customs of the day.[60]

Abortions

Abortions are not common to women in Malemia. Only two admitted they had an abortion.[61] One woman said it was while at secondary school in 1989. She was afraid that that would have been the end of her education. She now believes it was the work of the devil in her life.

> I took Surf foam, mixed it with some herbs and drank the liquid. I got very sick afterwards, but the teachers never noticed it was an abortion. So, I was safe. I was not yet a born again by then and the devil was working in me. But now I have received Jesus as my saviour. I am saved.[62]

The other woman said that she had not expected the baby to come that soon as she was still breastfeeding another. At St Luke's Hospital, the service providers admitted to receiving cases of abortions. That is why they encourage women to seek contraceptives so that a pregnancy should be by choice and not by chance.[63]

---

breech births and twins are considered as abnormal births. Breech delivery is when the baby starts coming out with buttocks first.

[60] Int. Woman 3, 9.1.2005. *Kale kunalibe mabvuto mukukumana nawo masiku anowa. Kunalibe kusanza, kudwaladwala ukakhala ndi mimba. Ngakhale pobereka sitimakumana ndi vuto lililonse. Ambiri amaberekera ku nyumba, pakhomo ndi a zamba. Osapeza vuto ata. Chifukwa chake, kusungamwambo.*

[61] This was one of the difficult questions posed. Despite enough probing, only these two admitted to have aborted.

[62] Int. N.N.

[63] Int. Matron, St Luke's Hospital, 18.1.2005.

Miscarriages

Having conceived, women feel joy and wait for the baby to come with so many expectations. A miscarriage is another terrible experience. Most women think miscarriage is normal and that there is nothing wrong with the mother. Most miscarriages happen in the first four months of the pregnancy. From my sample, 20 women representing 44 % have had a miscarriage or two. Most of those who had miscarried did so after an illness of some sort like malaria. Miscarriage is spontaneous. Some women think that miscarriages are a result of pressure from work.[64]

> I had a miscarriage in 2002 when the pregnancy was four months old. I went to the garden to farm when suddenly I felt my underwear getting wet. I thought I wanted to urinate and went to a nearby bush to help myself. It was there that I realized I was menstruating. I was rushed to Domasi Rural Hospital where they also referred me to Zomba Central Hospital for treatment. I had lost the pregnancy.[65]

Risky Sexual Reproductive Health Behaviour

Challenges of singlehood coupled with economic pressure force many women to indulge in risky behaviour. All women from my sample who admitted to such behaviour were unmarried. While most unmarried women said that they had abstained for a long time, waiting for a man who never seemed to come, a few said they no longer valued sexual intercourse and only did it for the sake of alleviating their poverty.

---

[64] It is normal for women to work long hours doing household chores regardless of their status, especially in rural areas. This is so because they do not have anyone to do the job. Thus, they do not have enough time to rest. In urban areas, the trend could be a bit different to some women who have a maidservant to help with the house chores.

[65] Int. Woman 4, 7.1.2005. I also recall my own experience when my pregnancy was two months old. One afternoon I realized I had started bleeding. I rushed to Zomba Central Hospital to see a gynaecologist. After scanning, the doctor told me it was a threatening abortion. But thank God he gave me some medication and prevented the miscarriage.

Below are some of these risky behaviours that may, in the long run, affect the sexual health of a woman.

Polygamy and Challenges of Singlehood

Polygamy seems to answer some of the challenges of singlehood.[66] The doctrine of the Islamic community allows polygamy where possible. In the time of the Prophet Muhammad when many men had died in war, leaving widows and children, the Prophet ordered that men could marry up to four wives to solve the problem of widowhood.

> If ye fear that ye shall not be able to deal justly with the orphans, marry women of your choice. Two, three, or four.[67]

In Malemia, polygamous marriages are not common. Extramarital affairs are again not frequent among married *women* from Malemia T/A.[68] Even most of those that are unmarried prefer to have one partner. Most women said it is degrading for a woman to have more than one partner and she can easily lose her reputation.[69]

---

[66] Among the women of this study, only one from the Muslim community is unmarried. A high percentage of unmarried women in this study are in the Christian community. Nevertheless, this is difficult to interpret. It does not necessarily mean it is a result of polygamy. There were, however, a few women from the Christian community who are married to Muslims.

[67] Quran Sura 4:3. This was after the battle of Uhud, when the Muslim community was left with many orphans and widows. Their treatment was governed by principles of humanity and equity.

[68] This was again another difficult question. To ask a married woman if she had extramarital affairs was so challenging. None from the sample amongst married women admitted to have an extramarital affair. Even if some may have had an affair besides their spouses, it was not possible to admit it for the sake of their own reputation. Still I trusted them as I do not have any evidence of any affairs. It is not that common according to our culture for married women to be moving around with boyfriends.

[69] For polygamy as Feminist challenge see: Moses Mlenga, *Polygamy in Northern Malawi. A Christian Reassessment*, Mzuzu: Mzuni Press, 2016, pp. 120-141. – Though Northern Malawi is mostly patrilineal, there are quite a number of aspects that apply also in matrilineal societies.

> At my age, where can I get a man of my age who is single to propose me? I also want a man.[70]

Most married women said that they know their husbands have extra-marital affairs. There is a wide perception amongst married women that their husbands have girlfriends. Only four women from the sample professed that they trust their husbands and know that they are the only ones for them. Some women said it is difficult to tell but still they do not trust their husbands to have only them as their wives. Women believe that polygamy in the church is not there in theory, but in practice it is evident. Or perhaps the appropriate term to use is risky behaviours. During Christianized *chinamwali*, promiscuity of girls is strongly condemned as evidenced from the following song.

Mtsikana woyendayenda, eeh!	The moving girl, eeh!
Mwana wafera panjira.	The child has died on the way.
Anafera panjira.	She died on the way.
Mwana wachigololo.	The fornicious child
Anafera panjira.	Died on the road.[71]

While widowhood affects both men and women, the heaviest burdens are borne by women. In many societies, including Malemia, it is easier to spot a woman who is unmarried than a man. The coming of HIV/Aids has affected the sexual and reproductive health of most women. "This pandemic has taken our men to the grave leaving us widows and children behind to look after."[72] Widowhood is a big challenge to women from Malemia Traditional Authority. The causes of singlehood

---

[70] Int. woman 14, 10.1.2005. *Kodi saizi yanga ino mnyamata oti angandi-funsire ndi mupeza kuti? Inenso ndimamufuna mwamuna. Chili kunzako umati chigwire nyanga.* The translation of the proverb is "if it is at someone else's (place), then you say grab it by the horns." Its meaning is that it is easy to blame other people for their mistakes or shortcomings while remaining blind to your own. Both translation and meaning taken from J.C Chakanza, *Wisdom of the People: 2000 Chinyanja Proverbs*, Blantyre: CLAIM-Kachere, 2000, p. 55.

[71] See Rachel NyaGondwe Fiedler, *Coming of Age. A Christianized Initiation among Women in Southern* Malawi, Zomba: Kachere, 2005, p. 73. She is referring to girls' initiation in a Baptist congregation.

[72] Int. N.N.

are widowhood and divorce, with widowhood in the lead. To be unmarried is common amongst women in Malemia. In my sample, the ratio of unmarried to married women is 5:7, which is not a big difference.

> I am a widow with many children and in order to feed the family, I have to buy three bags of maize a month. Those children at primary school are required to be paying K20 a month for development work. Where will I get the money? Of course, I have several partners, at times even three. When one gives me K200, another K150 and another K300, I find I have enough money to buy a bag of maize."[73]

Some of these unmarried women said they have passed the stage of enjoying sex and all they want is money. To these women, Malawian men are stingy and cannot just offer financial support free of charge.

> Nyere inatha kale kale. Sindimva chilichonse, amangwetu. Kumangodzumila chamkatikati, osawonetsera kuti ukunyansidwa kuti angasamuke. Iiii, ayi ndithu. Azibambo aku Malawi angakupatse ndalama yaulere osakugona, sizingatheke, amangwetu.[74]

---

[73] Int. N.N. The lady complains of her dire need for money. *Ine ndine wamasiye, amuna anga anamwalira, anandisiyira ana ambiri. Onsewa ndi adyetsa chiyani? Pamwezi ndimayenera ndigule matumba achimanga atatu, ana akupulayimale akufuna ma K20. Ndalama ndizitenga kuti? Ndizoonadi, zibwezizo zilipodi, nthawi zina ziwiri, zinthu zikavuta zitatu. Wina akakupatsa K150, wina K200, winanso K300. Basi thumba lachimanga lakwana* On challenges of singlehood, see also Rachel NyaGondwe Banda, *Women of Bible and Culture. Baptist Convention Women in Southern Malawi*, Zomba: Kachere, 2005, p. 188.

[74] Int. N.N. "I lost all my sexual desires long time ago. I do not feel anything, oh my friend! I just murmur quietly, without showing that I loath the sexual act for fear that he may leave. Oh, no! Malawian men, can they give you free money without sleeping with you, impossible, my friend!" The unfortunate thing is that these are not stable relationships. The so-called "boyfriends" are just temporary. Some relationships only last weeks before hunting for another man. Thus having more than one is not a big deal for these women as you are not so sure how long this one will last.

HIV/Aids or not, these unmarried women say they do not have any choice. Most do not even care about it. Condoms are rarely used and if used, not consistently.

> Today I can tell my boyfriend to put on a condom. And he can comply. Tomorrow I do the same, he complies again. The third day he will forget the condom deliberately and instead brings a plastic bag full of things like sugar, bread and soap. Are you going to refuse him sex because of a condom when there is no soap at home? It is not easy to do that. Then he will go back together with the bag."[75]

Remarriage

This is another challenge of being single. In this time of HIV/Aids, a divorcee or a widow is left in a dilemma of whether to marry again or to remain unmarried.[76] Unplanned remarriages in this time of HIV/Aids certainly may affect the sexual and reproductive health of a woman. None of those who have remarried thought about an HIV test before moving into the new home. Most women say, although it is a prere-

---

[75] Int. N.N. The literal translation is: *Lero umuwuza bvala kondomu, abvala, mawa bvala kondomu, abvala. Tsiku lachitatu ayiwalira dala satenga kondomu koma mmalo mwake abweretsa jumbo. Ukalandira jumbo ukana kugona naye poti alibe kondomu? Ndiye abwerera nayotu jumbo yakeyo. Ndiye iwe ukaganiza kunyumba kulibe shuga, sopo, basi uvulatu wekha, osawumulizidwa.*

[76] Rachel Banda comments that because it is difficult to find spouses that are free from HIV/Aids, some Baptist women who may desire to remarry opted to remain single (Rachel NyaGondwe Banda, *Women of Bible and Culture. Baptist Convention Women in Southern Malawi, Zomba: Kachere, 2005*, p. 189. It is however doubtful that these women indeed abstain faithfully, and then may they be praised. From my study, total abstinence seems to be a failure, even to those that are HIV positive. Most of these unmarried women are in their young ages. In such cases, I certainly believe that remarriage, whether you are HIV positive or not, is the best way out as long as both partners plan it beforehand and know their HIV status. On the other hand, I support fully the second observation of the Baptist women who are HIV positive and remain single for fear of endangering their lives. They fear the risk of bearing children that may also be HIV positive. This is very true. Even if you choose to remarry, pressure from your husband would force you to bear a child regardless of your status.

quisite to do so, knowing one's status is a difficult challenge. Fear of HIV/Aids surrounds all women. From my study, there are few remarriages in Malemia T/A. Only four women from the case study had remarried. From these four, one was a widow whose husband died three years ago. She married again in 2003.[77] The other three were divorcees.[78]

Contraception

Most women both married and unmarried go for contraceptives. Family planning is one of the health needs to most women. It is a key to greater health and prosperity.[79] The main reason for contraceptives to most women is to space rather than limit births. They want to rest from their birth experiences for a while. Although many women see the need for a small family, most would be happy if they bore five children. Five seems to be a big number. Most women opt for modern types of birth control. A very small percentage goes for traditional or natural methods. To many women, natural birth control does not always work and is not reliable.

> I go for modern type of method although my church objects to that. I tried the natural one and it failed. It was a complete blunder and many people thought I was careless when I had an emergency pregnancy when my baby was 10 months old. I can't do it again. I use pills.[80]

---

[77] Int. Woman 27, 13.1.2005.

[78] Int. Woman 24, 10.1.2005; Woman 17, 11.1.2005, Woman 5, 9.1.2005. The first woman says she left the husband on her own because the man was asking for her consent to bring a second wife into the home. The second woman left the first home because of the man's violence especially to do with sex. The third, who has two children from her first marriage, was divorced in 1995 and remarried in 1997. This marriage ended a year later when she was divorced again when the husband said he could not manage to feed her two children. She is now married to a third man.

[79] Gillian Paterson, *Love in a Time of AIDS: Women, Health and the Challenge of HIV*, Geneva: WCC, 1996, p. 6.

[80] Int. Woman 18, 11.1.2005.

Following the doctrines of the Catholic Church, a small percentage of women go for natural methods. They follow the calendar of their menstrual cycle and to some this works pretty well. One woman who respects her faith spoke as follows

> I go for what my Catholic church says. It encourages women to use natural birth control. Besides, I choose not to use modern ones because they have several side effects on one's health.[81]

Almost every woman is knowledgeable of contraceptives.[82] The hospital personnel gives enough and valuable knowledge to their clients. All women of reproductive age are welcome at St Luke's Hospital to seek

---

[81] Int. Woman 22, 17.1.2005. Compare sporadic abstinence in Ann K. Blanc et al, *Negotiating Reproductive Outcomes in Uganda, Kampala: Makerere University, 1996*. This is a unique method of preventing pregnancy by avoiding sexual intercourse through various means such as pretending to be ill, spending nights away from home or facing the wall (p. 35). On being asked whether they can manage this, most women from Malemia said this is impossible and not true. For comparative analysis see also, Garrett Hardin, *Birth Control*, New York: Pegasus, 1970. Hardin talks about the need for birth control through abortion and contraception. The author introduces the book by stating the tense atmosphere on contraceptives in the late 19th century. Tension against contraceptives came not only from the religious circle. In 1909, Father Arthur Vermeersch from Belgium published a document against contraceptives in which he emphasized strongly that it is the duty of a religious wife to dissuade her husband from using a condom and even to prefer rape to contraception (p. 21). On the same, Dr John Taylor, President of the British Gynaecological Society stated that family planning is evil. In his words, a family with only 2 or 3 children would be the downfall of the British Empire (p. 21).

[82] Emphasis was on types of contraceptives and their side effects. For comparative analysis, see Thomas Bisika et al, "Banja la Mtsogolo – Family Planning and STI Client Satisfaction Study", 2001, (no publisher). In their research, the authors observed that family planning clients are not always given full information about the full range of family planning services in the BLM clinics including their side effects (p. 10). The authors comment that one of the myths or rumours about family planning was that BLM is on a population control campaign and that some methods such as the pill lead to infertility.

contraceptives. There is no discrimination in relation to one's marital status, faith or age.[83]

> I will never buy a condom again. It is childish. I once bought Chishango condoms from a grocery to keep in my home that when my boyfriend comes he should use it. I will never do it again, I just wasted my money. He refused them saying that condoms give him tough time. I still cry for my K25. I could have bought *matemba* (small fish) for my children.[84]

On what happens to condoms that people buy from shops, some women said they did not know how they are used. Those married believe perhaps their partners use them to sleep with other women. One woman commented that they just put them on display and are thrown away after a time.

> I sought out condoms from the hospital one day when my husband was alive. Sister, it was a dispute. Frankly, he only used them for two days before saying, throw them away. I tried telling him I

---

[83] Int. Mrs Maloya, antenatal service provider, St Luke's, 19.01.2005. Every client is treated equally. Compare Hilda Saeed, "We Can't Stop Now: Pakistan and the Politics of Reproduction" in *Private Decisions, Public Debate: Women, Reproduction and Population,* 1994. Saeed disagrees with those who think that family planning is not Islamic. The author comments that Islam today is not as significant an obstacle to family planning as was once feared. Saeed believes that it is not only religious conservatism or lack of education that generate opposition to family planning, but also culture and one's attitude. To some people, having many children, especially sons, is a matter of honour, a sign of virility (p. 145). Hardin describes this concept as Machismo. Machismo is a Spanish word that implies masculinity. In Latin America, one important way a man demonstrates his manhood is by fathering many children. See Garrett Hardin, *Birth Control*, New York: Pegasus, 1970, p. 25.

[84] Int. Woman 43, 16.1.2005. *Sindidzagulanso ine kondomu. Mchibwana zedi. Ndinagulapo ine chishango ku golosale kumasunga mnyumba kuti chibwenzi changa chidzagwiritse ntchito. Ndithu, ndinangowononga ndalama yanga padera. Atakana ali zimenezi zimamutangwanikitsa. Ndikanaililabe K25 yanga mpaka pano. Ndikanagula matemba ana ndi kudya.*

become sick with pills but he said wear waist string. From that time, I never did it (seek condoms) again.[85]

But even unmarried women said that their partners do not use condoms. Sometimes they bring them and go away without using them. But most times they do not come with a condom and pretend to have forgotten it when asked for one by the partner.

> These things came late. It is a pity there is HIV/Aids otherwise we cannot manage using condoms. I once slept with my boyfriend. After everything that's when he realized he had a condom in the pocket of his trousers. He returned with it. Whether he used it with someone else, I don't know, perhaps he threw it away.[86]

At St Luke's, when a woman delivers she is advised to start family planning and resume sexual intercourse with her partner after six weeks. From 5601 clients at St Luke's, only three clients sought condoms totaling 18. See Table below for St Luke's 2004 records.

Family planning clients and type of methods sought from January to December 2004.

Injectables	5149	92%
Pill	434	8%
Condoms	3	0%
Others	15	0%
Total	5601	**100%**

---

[85] Int. Woman 45, 15.2.2005. *Ndinakatengapo makondomu kuchipatala tsiku lina ine mwamuna wanga ali moyo. Chemwali inali milandu. Ndithu anagwiritsa ntchito masiku awiri ali kataye. Ine kuyesera kuti mapilitsa wa amandidwalitsa, ali manga mkuzi. Kuchokera pomwepo sindinachitenso.* The husband died in 2003.

[86] Int. Woman 36, 16.1.2005. "*Zinthuzi zinabwera mochedwa. Yangovuta edzi makondomuwa sitingawathe. Ine ndinagonapo ndi chibwenzi changa. Zonse zitatha ndipamene amazindikira kuti anali ndi kondomu muthumba lathalauza. Mpaka anabwerera nayo, kaya anakagwiritsira ntchito kwina kaya, kaya anataya, hedeeeilii.*

> Those that go for family planning are the ones that have children. To me there is no reason for that because I do not have a child. Since 1999 when I got married up to now, a child is missing. I tried walking to traditional healers, not helping me. I know who bewitched me – my own relatives in Mangochi.[87]

Few churches encourage their members to plan their families.[88] However, even these do not specify the number of children per couple. That is left in the hands of the couple themselves, especially the husband, who is usually the one who decides how many children to have, usually without even considering economic factors. Few couples discuss the best family size. Even culture does not specify the number of children nor does it encourage parents to discuss it. In faith communities, the issue of family size and contraceptives is not discussed and considered openly. From my sample, none of the women reported to have received any advice from their faith communities on the need for family planning. Most churches such as CCAP and SDA are quiet on family planning.[89]

Women and Condom Use

Most women interviewed said they would be happy to use condoms whether for contraception or HIV/Aids prevention. To enjoy sexual intercourse depends for them on the skill of both the man and the

---

[87] Int. Woman 1, 8.1.2005. Born 1970 and married in 1999, this woman cannot conceive. *Amene amalera ndi amene ali ndi ana. Kwa ine palibe chifukwa cholelera poti mwana ndilibe. Chikwatiwileni 1999 mpakana pano mwana akundisowa. Ndayesa kuyenda mwa a sing'anga osathandiza. Ndimadziwa amene anandilodza—abale anga omwe aliku Mangochi.* Compare Jean Garland, *Aids is Real and it's in our Church, Bukuru: African Christian Textbooks, 2003*, p. 148. Garland comments that one of the harmful traditions relating to sex is that the ancestors curse those women who do not conceive. The author believes that this false belief may cause Aids to spread in such that childlessness may be used as an excuse for sexual intercourse outside marriage.

[88] Such churches include Roman Catholic and Pentecostal churches. Int. Woman 14. However, those who reported this emphasized that what is discussed is not the family size but the type of contraceptives to choose.

[89] Int. Woman 7, 10.1.2005 and Woman 3, 9.1.2005.

woman and not because one is not wearing a condom. Those that had once used a condom said they did not find any difference in pleasure between sex with a condom and sex without. All is the same.

> I do not see any difference. Although men say with a condom sex is not enjoyable, that is not true. It is that such people are not expert in bed. Do not blame a condom. Even eating sweets with a wrapper is still sweet. The moment you just put it in your mouth, you may not feel the sweetness. But once you start sucking it, you even reach a point that you forget that you are sucking together with a wrapper. Sometimes, swallowing the sweet together with the wrapper.[90]

Unfortunately, despite their wish, women both married and unmarried do not use condoms. All women interviewed said they do not because of pressure from their partners who seem not to like them either. It can be concluded that almost no one is using a condom. In the Christian society, those that are married have an advantage on condom over the unmarried, in the sense those churches that accept a condom do so only at the marriage level.[91] Married women believed that an unmarried woman is better off at negotiating condom use from her partner than someone who is married. They believed that unmarried women have greater power than married ones to refuse their partners sex without a condom and are at a greater advantage of avoiding HIV/Aids if at all a condom is reliable and can prevent HIV/Aids.

> A boyfriend can entice you if you are his girlfriend. He can respect your desire and put on a condom for fear of losing you. A girlfriend

---

[90] Int. Woman 26, 15.1.2005. *"Ine ndiye sindimawona kusiyana kwake. Ngakhale azibambowa amavuta kuti ati ndi kondomu sizikoma, bodza. Kumangokhala kusaidziwa ntchitoyo, osanamizira kondomu. Ingakhale suwiti yodyera mpepala, moti siikoma? Mwina ukangoponyamo kumene mkamwamo koma ukangoukulumunya pang'ono umafikanso pena kuyiwala kuti ukudya ndichipepala chomwe. Kutsala pang'ono kumeza ndipepala lomwe kuli kukoma."*

[91] Married women have support from some churches over condom use whether it be used as a contraceptive or as a device for HIV/Aids prevention. Christian churches do not encourage unmarried women to use condoms as that would be promiscuity.

has all the freedom to dump the man and find another. But not in marriage. He can just tell you that that is the end of the marriage. Go and find the one who has no HIV virus. I will get another wife. It is difficult to a married wife.[92]

The above remark was however contradicted when I interviewed the unmarried if at all this chance is there. To them it is the married who can encourage their husbands to use condoms, not the singles. They believed marriage is a stable relationship and such things can be discussed openly and not in loose relationships.

A boyfriend today, we entice him in order that he should come again tomorrow. You cannot tell a boyfriend what to do. He will leave you and go to someone else. If he wants the condom he will use it. If he does not, he cannot. A girlfriend has no power over that. If he leaves you, where will you go? Do you just have to be moving around looking for men like hyenas from Ntcheu? It is better in marriage; a wife is given some respect. A marriage does not just end anyhow. Divorce because of a condom issue? It can't happen. Of course, there are also some women who do not like a condom. They say skin to skin. It is a pity I am failing to find a marriage partner. I cannot allow sleeping with my husband without a condom when I know for sure that he is promiscuous. He would be putting on a condom and the marriage will continue. Unless he had another reason for divorcing me.[93]

---

[92] Int. Woman 9, 10.1.2005. *Chibwenzi chimanyengerera chingathe kukumvera ndi kuvala kondomu powopa kuti uli ndi ufulu onse kumusiya kukapeza china chibwenzi. Koma osati pabanja. Angokuuza kuti basi lathera pomwepa banja pitani kapezeni opanda edziwo. Ine ndipeza wina mkazi. Ndizovuta na mzimayi wa pabanja.*

[93] Int. Woman 8, 10.1.2005. *Afisi aku Ntcheu* was a popular song a few years ago. Sung by notable musician, Joseph Nsaku, the song had a message about unmarried women who go around aimlessly looking for men like hyenas. During this time, hyenas had given tough time to the people in Ntcheu. This was the reason for his reference to Ntcheu district. *Chibwenzi masiku ano timachita kunyengerera, mkonya patali patali kuti abwerenso mawa. Chibwenzi siungachiuze chochita, chikusiya chiyendera ina. Ngati akufuna kondomuyo, avala yekha, ngati sakufuna savala. Koma iwe ulibe mphamvu yomuuza*

Women have no power to use condoms. In most societies including Malemia, it is not acceptable for a married woman to ask her husband to use a condom. Most women said their men would call them "hule" (prostitute).[94] A few from the unmarried group said they use it sometimes, but it is just occasional. These women again said they cannot put a condom on their partner because it is embarrassing for a woman to do that.[95] None of the women reported to have used condoms consistently. One woman commented that it depends on the mood that day and it is as if they just dreamt about it all of a sudden.

> We used it twice when we were just starting our relationship. After that we got used to each other and we have sexual intercourse without a condom. What else could I have done? During the second time, I made up my mind to be using condoms. I went to the hospital to see a sick friend. She had grown thin like this child of mine. It touched my heart and I told myself to be keeping condoms. On this day, I was also lucky because my boyfriend had just quarrelled with

---

zochita. Akakusiya upita kuti? Uzingokhalira yambakata yambakata mumseu kufuna amuna ngati afisi aku Ntcheu. Bola mbanja, mkazi amakupatsako ulemu. Banja silimangotha chisawawa. Kutha chifukwa chakondomu? Sizinga-chitike, alipoto azimayi ena nawonso samasangalatsidwa ndi kondomu. Ati thupi ku thupi. Ine likungondisowa ndibanjalo, sindingalore kugona ndimwa-muna wanga wambanja opanda kondomu nditamuvera mbiri kuti ali ndi zibwenzi. Avala basi banjanso osatha, maseweratu, ndiye anali ndichifukwa ndikale.

[94] This term depicts a bad message as well on condoms. It is as if everyone that uses them does so in an unacceptable way. Most women also commented that partners rebuke them at the mentioning of condoms, asking them whether they think they (the men) are HIV positive. Compare Suwanna Asavaroengchai, "Double Standard Double Threat: HIV and Reproductive Health in Thailand" in *Private Decisions, Public Debate: Women, Reproduction and Population*, London: Panos, 1994. The author agrees that condom is a sensitive issue for marital sex. Even if well informed about HIV and how it is spread, wives rarely discuss safer sex with husbands who have other partners. Usually the topic of condoms ends in blows (p. 114).

[95] On how to use a condom, see Pakachere booklet, p. 5.

his wife over family issues. So, he had no choice but to put on a condom as I had wanted for fear of dying twice.[96]

Women can do little, even to protect themselves, as in most homes the man seems to be in charge of condom use. There is also an attitude in this society that condoms are for those that are HIV positive.[97] Most women believe when you know you are HIV positive, it is very easy to negotiate condom use and even your partner can understand that.

Women and Sexual Intercourse

While some women said that they do not like sex, others said they cannot do without it. For most of the women, sexual intercourse leads to pleasure and enrichment of the family life. Sexual life in most homes and to most women is a prerequisite. Many women expressed the same sentiments that it is strange that if the marriage is newly fresh, the love is also strong and sex is frequent, but when a woman gives birth for the first time, the love starts dying slowly.[98] Most women, especially those married, have sex, even thrice a day and get surprised when they hear their husbands have partners outside.

> We do not know what men want when they go out for other women. I do not think it is sex because we give them sex anytime

---

[96] Int. Woman 26, 15.1.2001. *Tinagwiritsirako ntchito kawiri kokha basi titangoyamba kumene chibwenzi chimenechi. Kenako tinazolowerana timangopanga basi opanda. Nanga ine ndiye nditani? Nthawi yachiwiriyo ndinalimba mtima kuti ndizigwiritsa ntchito kondomu. Ndinapita kuchipatala kukawona mzanga akudwala, atawonda ngati mwana wangayu. Ndinakhu-dzidwa ndati basi ndizikhala ndi kondomu. Mwayi wakenso tsiku limeneli akuti anali atakangana ndi mkazi wake kunyumba kwake, nkhani zawo zambanja. Ndiye analibenso matukutuku koma kuvala basi kuopa kufa kuwiri.*

[97] Perhaps it is due to the fact that condoms became widely known in Malawi with the arrival of HIV/Aids. Thus most women from this area believe that the advent of condoms is associated with the virus. In this way, if you are free from the virus, you are also free from condom use. The messages that are depicted in Malawi on condom use to avoid HIV/Aids, have created a negative implication on condoms.

[98] Int. Woman 16, 11.1.2005.

they want. Even when you are cooking, they can call you to leave your *nsima* on the fire. We comply and give them. But still they will walk away.[99]

Fear of HIV/Aids has affected the attitude of women to sex. Most women said sexual intercourse today is not pleasant, not in a sense that women do not enjoy it, but fear destroys the whole mood. However, despite this fear, sex is, to many, a priority. They cannot abandon sexual life because of HIV/Aids.

Sexual intercourse today is not pleasant due to mistrust and fear of HIV/Aids. We just do it because it is nature.[100]

There is no specific time for sex in many homes. It is done whenever the desire comes. However, in most homes, it is usually in the evening when children are asleep and when the woman is resting from her daily house chores or early in the morning. This is why at *chinamwali*, initiates are told not to go to their parents' bedroom in the morning.

In the morning, if you go to your mother's house, you will find the penis in the vagina.[101]

Most women have sex in the dark when the lamp is off. This is not only because of embarrassment to see each other's private parts but also to respect sex. A few reported of not being ashamed at all with one's body but that it is simply to save paraffin.

Sometimes we have sex three times during the night. Can we manage to make love with the lamp on? Everything is expensive

---

[99] Int. Woman 8, 10.1.2005. Because almost all these women are housewives, it is easy to have sex in this way. They spend their times at home.

[100] Int. Woman 7, 10.1.2005. *Kugonana masiku ano sikukukoma, kukayikilana, nkhawa basi kuti mwina ndilinako kapena mzangayu. Timangochitira poti ndi chilengedwe.*

[101] The text is taken from Patrick Makondesa, "Initiation Rites in Southern Malawi and Related Territories", MA, Module 1, p. 5. *Mmawamawa kwa amayi udzapeza malikitiki mbolo ili ng'ang'ang'a Nyini.*

these days including paraffin. So, to have sex in the dark is not necessarily because we are ashamed to be seen by the husband but rather to save paraffin. Sometimes we do not have the paraffin at all. Should we spend the little money we have for that?[102]

Still, non-sexual nakedness is not common in the area. Although a few women said they can and do at times bathe with their husbands, most felt it is not appropriate. They feel embarrassed to do so. Some women said they even feel ashamed to dress in the presence of their husbands. One woman refuted this to be associated with initiation teachings. She spoke as follows.

There is nothing wrong with exposing your nakedness to your husband. The church teaches us that marriage is one body and there is no need to be embarrassed with one another. In my church, we have marriage seminars where such issues are discussed.[103]

In many homes, talking about sexual matters continues to be seen as a taboo. In Malemia T/A, though their culture is a bit flexible and not very strict in sexual matters, it is still not easy for a woman to introduce the subject to her partner. Women play a small role in sexual life; men are dominating as they are the ones that engineer sex. Most women feel embarrassed to talk about sex with their husbands.

Where can you start from? It is not proper for a woman to do that. You give your husband a bad picture. Stories on lovemaking are not something you can ask your husband. Why don't you ask your fellow woman? What he wants he will let you know. You just have

---

[102] Int. Woman 4, 7.1.2005.

[103] Int. Woman 3, 1.6.2005. *Palibe cholakwika kuwonetsa umaliseche wako munthu kwa mwamuna wako. Ku mpingo amatiwuza kuti banja ndi thupi limodzi sipafunika kuchitilana manyazi. Ku mpingo kwathu timakhalaso ndi maphunziro a banja kumene izi zimakambidwanso.* This woman belongs to SDA. At such seminars, unmarried women (those that have been married before such as widows and divorcees) are invited to attend. Both groups sit together. Marriage seminars in SDA churches take place once a year.

to obey. Besides, where will you find that spare time to talk about that?[104]

Only few women felt free to discuss sex with their husbands. These few women said that they can ask their men to make love to them though this is not always easy. However, if words fail, they do it through actions by touching the man's genitals. When satisfied with sex, most women are happy and free to congratulate their partners. This is not the case when they are not. Most remain quiet and pretend all is well. Very few women are free to tell their partners how they feel about sex, if at all they enjoy it or not.

> I can tell my partner how I am feeling about it, whether I have enjoyed it or not. I can tell him to start again when I feel not satisfied. If I am ashamed to him, who else will I talk to? He is my husband and I love him. Love experiences no shame.[105]

Most women said that if they initiate sex, their husbands accuse them of having an affair with another man and call her a prostitute. It is rare for women to initiate sex even if they have the desire for it. Culturally, a woman should wait for the man to start the game. From my study, some women too felt that men are solely responsible for initiating sex.

---

[104] Int. Woman 24, 14.1.2005. *Uyambira pati. Siulemu mkazi kumachita zime-nezo. Umamupatsa chithunzi thunzi choipa mwamuna. Nkhani zogonana ndi zosati ukhale pansi uzifunsa mwamuna siulemu. Osakafunsa mkazi mzako bwanji? Zimene akufuna iyeyo akuwuza. Iwe kwako ndi kumvera. Ndiponso ndi nthawi yokambirana zimenezoyo uyitenga kuti?*

[105] Int. Woman 22, 13.1.2005. *Ndingathe kumuuza kuti sizikukoma kapena ndi kukomedwa. Kaya sizinayende ayambirenso. Kuti bambo mwangokhetsa thu-kuta lopanda phindu, palibe ndiona ine heheee. Ndikachita manyazi kumuuza ndiye ndikauzanso ndani? Ndi mwamuna wanga kaya ndimakukondani. Chikondi chilibe manyazi.*

A woman has no power to do that. Is she a prostitute or is she sexy? It is a man that should ask for sex because he is the one who proposed you.[106]

During initiation of *Chiputu*, songs teach that women should not ask sex from men. The man should desire it by himself. One such song is the one below.[107]

Song 4

Mwana mnyamata usagone.	Young man, do not sleep.
Utogona?	Are you sleeping?
Ona dina.	See my vagina.
Tandileke, tandileke.	Leave me, leave me alone.
Ndamwa mowa.	I drank beer.

Because of this cultural perception that a man is responsible for sex, some married women feel that their husbands do not want sex from them and disappoint them whenever they engineer sexual intercourse. They added that sometimes their own husbands embarrass them in public once they dare do that. This is why they normally choose to remain quiet and wait for the man to start it.

My husband embarrassed me one day when he was telling his friends at a beer hall that I like sexual intercourse. Saying, do not just see that woman. She likes it. She is always sexy and continuously asking for sex like a prostitute.[108]

---

[106] Int. Woman 10, 10.1.2005. *Mkazi alibe mphamvu, ndi hule, ali ndi nyere? Mwamuna ndi amene amakufuna kuti akugone, amene anakufunsira, kutatukura ku moyo.*

[107] Taken from *Coming of Age*, p. 74. In the song, the wife shows her husband her vagina. The man refuses saying he has just taken beer and is tired. The meaning is to show that a woman must not ask for sexual intercourse.

[108] *Ndinayalukapo ine amuna anga akumawauza anthu kumowa kuti ine ndimakonda chigololo. Ati; musamangomuona mkazi amene uja, amaziko-ndatu, nyere pafupi pafupi, kuchita kufunsa ngati hule.* This was a comment from a member from the Anglican Church during group discussions at Mpira prayer house on 30.1.2005. According to Steven Paas, *Chichewa-Chinyanja*

46

All women commented that knowledge of sexual life in a family is totally in the hands of the couples. When they come under one roof, they are solely responsible for that. However, some churches aid the couple with "bedroom instructions". In Christian initiation rites, it is commonly known as *chilangizo*. They differ at a very marginal point with that done traditionally.[109] Although not detailed to include sex styles, most women that had undergone these bedroom instructions appreciated them.[110] The day before the wedding day, both the groom and the bride receive some *mwambo* (instructions) on how they are to go about sexual intercourse. Unfortunately, from my study, not many women had their weddings in the church. Most women relied on their traditional initiation ceremonies. During *chinkhoswe*, there is not much instruction given on sexual life. What is said is mainly to be committed and faithful to each other until the wedding day. One woman who underwent chinkhoswe said:

> There was not much said on sexual life as such. What the instructors emphasized was faithfulness. They advised us that this was not a wedding per se but just an engagement. We were asked to break with any other relationships if we had any since we are now committed to each other. As a lady, I was advised to be committed to my prospective husband and never to be moved by some men who may come to me with money.[111]

English Dictionary, chigololo is translated as adultery, fornication and coitus. In this context, it refers to sexual intercourse with the wife.

[109] For details on initiation rites in the Church, refer to Rachel NyaGondwe Banda, *Women of Bible and Culture: Baptist Convention Women in Southern Malawi*, Zomba: Kachere, 2005. See also Molly Longwe, *From Chinamwali to Chilangizo: The Christianization of Pre-Christian Chewa Initiation Rites in the Baptist Convention of Malawi*, MA, University of Natal, Pietermaritzburg, 2003.

[110] On the real wedding day, emphasis is again placed on sexual life that none should refuse each other sex. Reference is mainly from the book of Genesis and 1st Corinthians 7. On types of marriages, see Rachel NyaGondwe Banda, *Women of Bible and Culture. Baptist Convention Women in Southern Malawi*, Zomba: Kachere, 2005, pp. 172-176.

[111] Int. Woman 31, 24.1.2005. Unfortunately, the instruction on faithfulness until marriage did not pay them at all. Before the wedding day, they had already

One CCAP woman who underwent *mwambo* on bedroom instructions during her wedding spoke as follows.

> It was Thursday, two days before my wedding day. The clock ticked 10:30 pm. The *mwambo* still continued. I was now getting bored and tired but I had no choice. Three counsellors, together with my aunt and a grandmother to my husband, were there. I had brought the items as requested. These were a plastic pail, a one-meter cloth, four small pieces of cloth plus a shaver. At around 8:00 pm, the *mwambo* had started. One woman in her deep voice spoke vigorously on the use of the items. The four small pieces were to be used to clean our private parts after each sexual intercourse. The long cloth was to be spread on the bed during the game to avoid wetting the beddings. The pail was for washing the items, the shaver for shaving private parts. After her came a man. He emphasized on foreplay and how to arouse each other in bed. One woman actually took hold of my husband's finger demonstrating it as a penis. I was told to rouse my husband by playing with the tip of it. My darling was also told to do the same.[112]

In addition to this, women stated that in their faith communities, they are told to obey the husband because he is the head of the family while men are to love their wives. During initiation, most women commented that in the past during *chinamwali,* some *namkungwi* could demonstrate a little bit how to do sex through songs and dance.[113] Most women said that it is still difficult even if you, the lady, were told this; most men do not know much about sex.[114] Besides, because of culture,

---

impregnated each other. Still, they are living together and have blessed their marriage from the same church.

[112] Int. Woman 6, 9.1.2005. This church was CCAP in the Blantyre Synod. For comments on bedroom instructions, see Fulata Moyo, "How to be Sexually Sexy—the Church Way: The Case of the Bedroom Instructions", paper presentation on instructions given at traditional weddings.

[113] Most songs are sung while the girls wriggle their waists. For details, see Rachel NyaGondwe Fiedler, *Coming of Age. A Christianized Initiation among Women in Southern* Malawi, Zomba: Kachere, 2005.

[114] It was however difficult to tell whether this lack of knowledge had directly to do with their initiation rites because boys too do get initiated or that some

most women, even if they know a little, cannot dare to tell their husbands.

> My husband behaves as if it is a fight. It is unfortunate to go into marriage and realize that your partner is not that good at sex. You cannot say anything for this could not be appropriate. Besides, he would ask you where you learnt the sex styles thinking you have extra marital affairs.[115]

All women said the support they get from their churches is encourage- ment to have only one sexual partner. Most women said that church doctrines are against adultery. This is regularly preached in the church.[116]To many women, this is a necessary doctrine, but not easy to follow. Most women say it is unfortunate that most people commit adultery but only that it is difficult to catch them. A woman is at a disadvantage because if she is careless and does not use contraceptives, she will be caught easily once she is pregnant. The penalty is the same in most churches: discipline for a certain period, which varies according to church. In CCAP, one undergoes a six months' discipline before being called to a church session. This is like a church court.[117] Most women said this punishment cannot stop many from becoming pregnant. Of course, as one woman commented, it is degrading to a

---

men do shun these rites. Isabel Phiri comments that boys are not told such things (*Women, Presbyterianism and Patriarchy. Religious Experience of Chewa Women in Central Malawi*, Blantyre: CLAIM-Kachere, 1997, p. 40). Patrick Makondesa too, in his module, never showed that boys are taught sexual techniques.

[115] Int. Woman 30, 18.1.2005. *Ine amuna anga amangokhala ngati nkhondo. Koma ndizovuta makamaka munthu ukakwatiwa ndikukapeza kuti bambo sizenizeni. Chili chibwenzi uchisiya, koma banja utuluka bwanji? Siunganeneso chilichonse, ndi mwano. Ndiponso akufunsa kuti zokomazo unazidziwira kuti? Nanga masitayilowo unawawonera kuti? Umagona ndi amuna ena eti?*

[116] Not to commit adultery is one of the Ten Commandments given to Moses at Mount Sinai. In some churches this preaching from Exodus 20 happens regularly to remind the whole congregation of good moral conduct.

[117] Part of the discipline is not to partake in the Eucharist.

woman to answer such charges amongst the clergy; however, they said they do not have a choice.

> I have two children out of wedlock. When I went again to the church session after my second child, the clergy shouted at me. Saying I am disrespectful, not even embarrassed to do it again for the second time. But what else could I have done?[118]

It is not common for couples to talk about their sexual lives. For some women, this is probably due to lack of time. Most women spend their time looking after their home and children. They spend no time chatting with their husbands. Some churches do at times conduct marriage seminars where couples can go and talk about sexual life. Those that have marital problems are encouraged to attend. In CCAP, this kind of seminar comes once a year. Only those married are to attend such seminars. Unmarried women such as widows and divorcees cannot attend because you have to go together with your spouse. One woman explained as follows the marriage seminar she attends in her church.

> When we arrive, we sit next to our husbands. We are counselled that marriage is one body therefore we should not fear each other. Do not hide anything from your partner. If something is amiss, discuss with your partner amicably. We are also told to sleep naked. There are some men who sleep with their trousers. When they want to start the job, they just take the penis carefully and put it back in the trouser after the job is over. These things should not happen. Wives are also told not to sleep with their petticoat or their underwear. There are some women who are difficult that even when their husbands tear the underwear, they will put on another pant. This should not happen in married life. There are some indeed with difficult marriages. Every day the man saying I am tired with office work. What about family job? Is marriage over? Here a wife should indeed mistrust her husband.

> Where is he getting tired and who is making him tired? Perhaps he has a girlfriend that is making him tired. Counsellors advise that

---

[118] Int. Woman 42, 15.3.2005. *Ine ndili ndi ana awiri amuchigololo. Anandinena kumilandu nthawi yachiwiriyi. Ali amayi inu ndinu osamva, ochititsa manyazi, mpaka kawiri. Koma nanga ndikanatani?*

when you the woman reach this stage of mistrust, play it cool. There are some women who become so angry to the extent of refusing to sleep with the man. As a wife, sit with your husband, ask him in a gentle manner. Remind him that there is a new disease in our land called HIV/Aids.[119]

Sex and Faith

There is a relationship between sex and faith in most Malawian societies including Malemia. Almost each woman in this area belongs to a particular faith. Malemia comprises two different faiths groups, Christianity and Islam. Both communities support their members in one

---

[119] Int. Woman 29, 18.1.2005. *Tikafika aliyense amayenera akhale pafupi ndi mwamuna wake. Amatilangiza kuti banja ndi thupi limodzi choncho tisamawopane. Osamabisa kanthu kukhosi ngati china chalakwika kambiranani mwa chikondi monga banja. Amatilangizanso kuti pogona ali yense azivula zovala. Alipo amuna ena amagona ndi thalauza lomwe, ikayamba ntchitoyo kungotulutsira momwemo, mukatha nkubwezeretsanso muthalauza momwemo. Izi amati zisamachitike. Ngakhale azimayi amatiwuzanso kuti tisamagone ndi pitikoti kapena panti. Alipo azimayi ena ovuta olo mwamuna akung'ambire panti, kuvalanso wina. Izinso zisamachitike mbanja. Alipodi mabanja ena amavuto. Mwamuna tsiku lililonse kumangoti ndatopa ku ntchito. Kodi ntchito ikhala ya ku ofesi yokha, mnyumba muno banja latha. Pamenepo iwe mkazi umayenera kukayika. Akutopa kuti, akumutopetsayo ndani. Umakayika kuti mwina ali ndi chibwenzi penapake ndi amene akumutopetsayo. Azilangizi amatifotokozera kuti mkazi ukafika poti wayamba umukayikira mwamuna wako, usachite phuma. Azimayi ena amafika pokana ndi kuchipinda komwe ati kukwiya. Mwamuna umunyengerere ndithu ngati mwana ndi kumufunsa mwa mtendere. Kuti amunanga kunja kuno kwayipa kuli matenda. Ukalakhula mwachikondi mwamuna amamva.* This church is CCAP. Other churches include Anglican and SDA. I wished I could attend a marriage seminar in February 2005. This was at my church, Domasi Jeanes CCAP. However as someone without a husband, I thought I should not dare go. I remembered how a friend in Lilongwe was actually pulled out of a certain church under the Synod of Nkhoma, when it was discovered that she was unmarried. I was however surprised that a friend who is unmarried attended this seminar at Jeanes. I don't know how she got there and what tricks she used. I think, Blantyre Synod is a bit flexible or perhaps no one realized that she is unmarried.

way or another. Although most women admitted that there is little support from their faith communities as regards their sexual reproductive health, belonging to a religion matters in a woman's life.

> A woman is kept busy with church work. She has no time to back-bite. She has no time to move aimlessly sleeping with someone's husband. What she does is cheering the sick, and praying and days just pass by.[120]

Women and HIV and Aids

Most women seem to be knowledgeable about HIV/Aids, how it is transmitted and what preventative measures there are. Many women said the best way to prevent HIV is to abstain and be faithful to your partner and when this fails, then use a condom. HIV/Aids is not often mentioned in churches. Sometimes this is mentioned only when there is a conference.

> Talking about HIV/Aids is not common in churches. At times, it is mentioned during conferences. We hear messages on HIV/Aids from the hospital and from the radio. Even in schools, children tell us that some people came to talk about HIV/Aids, but not in the church, it is seldom.[121]

A few women felt HIV/Aids is *kanyera*.[122] *Kanyera* is an illness that attacks both the child and the father. A newborn child could be born

---

[120] Int. Woman 7, 10.1.2005. *Mzimayi amatangwanika ndi za mpingo. Nthawi yochitira miseche alibe. Nthawi yoyenda yenda kumagona ndi amuna a eni ake alibenso. Iye zake basi ndi kucheleza anthu odwala, kupemphera, basi masiku mkumapita hedeeeee ilii.*

[121] Int. Woman 3, 9.1.2005. *Sikwenikweni kutchula zamatendawa mtchalichi. Nthawi zina kumisonkhano yamisasa amatha kunena. Za edzi timazimvera kuchipatala kapena muwailesi. Ngakhalenso kusukulu ana amatiwuza kuti kunabwera odzanena za edzi, koma osati ku tchalichi ayi, ndi panthawi.* Some churches do have annual conferences. In SDA, they are commonly known as *misasa*.

[122] For details on Kanyera see Rachel NyaGondwe Fiedler, *Coming of Age. A Christianized Initiation among Women in Southern* Malawi, Zomba: Kachere, 2005, p. 86. "Chinyela, chinyela/ chitha amuna/ Akazi natsala."

with *kanyera* and men are required to follow the cultural practice of sexual abstinence towards the wife during a certain period to avoid *kanyera*.

> There is no escape; HIV/Aids is there too in the church. The adultery is coming from the very church. Most of us pretend to be holy when we are in the church but once we come out, we are different. A religion that is being put on like clothes. Every day, making confessions to the priest on the same sin.[123]

A few women commented that HIV/Aids is a plague that was prophesied long time ago in the Old Testament. There is nothing that a woman can do as this is just fulfilling what God said.

> You just have to stay. Waiting patiently for the day when the virus will find you. What else can you do? This is a plague. God said that He would send a wasting disease to those that are disobedient. Is this not HIV/Aids?[124]

---

[123] Int. Woman 17, 11.1.2005. *Palibe pothawira, mumpingo edziyo ilipo, chigololocho chi kuchokera mumpingo momwemo. Ambiri tikalowa mchalichi timawoneka ngati achiyere. Tikangotuluka, zonse zathera momwemo. Timabvalanso zina zobvala. Chipembedzo chochita kuvala. Daily kulapa kwa a nsembe machimo ake amodzimodzi.*

[124] Int. Woman 3, 9.1.2005. *Basi kungokhala. Kumangodikira kuti kaya iwe kakupeza liti kachilomboka. Nanga nkutani? Ndimuliri uwu. Mulungu ananena kuti kwa onse osamvera ndidzatumiza matenda owondetsa. Nanga si edziyi?* – The woman believes HIV/Aids is a "wasting disease" (*matenda owondetsa)* as recorded in the book of Leviticus 26:16 in which God was telling his people the Israelites the punishment that would befall them if the disobeyed Him. The Chichewa translation of Leviticus 26:16 reads: "...ndidzachitira inu icinso; ndidzakuikirani zoopsa, nthenda yoondetsa ya m'chifuwa ndi malungo, zakulanda maso ndi mphamvu, ndi kuzunza moyo..."(Buku Lopatulika). The English translation is: "...then I will do this to you: I will bring upon you a sudden terror, wasting diseases and fever that will destroy your sight and drain away your life..."(NIV). This passage is used by many people including some members of the clergy in many Christian churches to refer to HIV/Aids as a plague prophesied thousands of years ago. Certainly the signs of this disease could be related to those of HIV/Aids. But to conclude that HIV/Aids is a plague could be misleading. Perhaps it is true, perhaps not, maybe this plague had already

To add to this comment, some women stressed the fact that it is their church that teaches them that HIV/Aids is a punishment from God to those that commit adultery. To most women, it is circumstances that force them to commit such sins. If the church encourages fidelity and one sexual partner, most married women say they can obey this commandment, but will their spouses do the same as well? To many women, it is difficult to measure faithfulness. Thus, even if you, a woman, are truly saved, if you are under the roof of a promiscuous husb

and, you cannot escape HIV/Aids.

> A married woman receives respect. It is better to marry and let the virus find you inside marriage and not outside. It is embarrassing to an unmarried woman to be HIV positive as if you were promiscuous.[125]

A few women counteract with the statement that it is better today to remain unmarried. To them, a single woman has a greater chance of initiating safe sex than a married woman, and therefore is able to save herself from HIV/Aids. Some women again commented that HIV is transmitted in several ways and not only through sex. As such there is still a chance of getting it through other ways when you have been truly faithful to your commandments.

> Religion cannot save a person from HIV. There are a number of ways how one contracts the virus including injections.[126]

Although it is not easy to escape HIV/Aids, faith is crucial to a woman in this context of HIV. A woman with faith has hope in Jesus. God teaches that he is the healer of all diseases; a woman who is religious is able to pray to God to heal her when she happens to be HIV positive.

---

happened. Nevertheless, it does not matter. HIV/Aids is HIV/Aids, whether a plague or not.

[125] Int. Woman 20, 12.1.2005. *Mayi wapabanja amalandira ulemu. Kuli bwino kukwatiwa kachilomboko ukakapezere m'banja osati kunja kwa banja. Zimachititsa manyazi ukaitengera kunja ngati kuti siumayenda bwino.*

[126] Int. Woman 27, 13.1.2005. *Chipembedzo sichingapulumutse munthu ku Edzi. Matendawa amabwera munjira zosiyanasiyana. Kuphatikizapo jakisoni.*

I once heard that some HIV positive people were healed after being prayed for.[127]

Some women said that in this time of HIV/Aids, a prayerful woman has the duty to pray for the life of her husband as well, so that he is faithful to her alone, and also to be a true born again.[128] A woman can be saved from the HIV Aids epidemic if she is faithful and religious. The fear of hell and even church discipline saves many women from death.

A church can save a woman from HIV/Aids. Fear saves. Fear of the church and the pastor makes one conscious not to be found in bad

places. Again, fear of being disciplined by the church once you have broken the church doctrines of committing adultery, can make a woman faithful to her husband, and avoid HIV.[129]

HIV/Aids and Witchcraft

The phenomenon of witchcraft is not very popular in this vicinity. There is no connection between witchcraft and HIV/Aids according to respondents from Malemia. From the sample, the majority of women denied that HIV infection is related to witchcraft. However, a few women commented that in some cases, some individuals who practice

---

[127] Int. Woman 22, 13.1.2005. *Ine ndinamvapo kuti anthu ena amene anapezeka ndi kachilomboka, anachira atapemphereredwa.* The woman however says she does not know who this person healed from HIV is because she just heard the story. However, she is certain that the story is true. The healed lady belongs to a Pentecostal church. – For a discussion of different healing claims see: Klaus Fiedler, *Fake Healing Claims for HIV/AIDS: Traditional, Christian and Scientific*, Mzuzu: Mzuni Press, 2016.

[128] Int. Woman 21, 12.1.2004. In the gospel of John, Jesus assured Nicodemus that no one would see the kingdom of God unless he is born again (John 3:3). There are so many people today who claim to be born again. But to find a "true" born again is another issue.

[129] Int. Woman 29, 18.1.2005. *Mpingo ungamupulumutse mzimayi ku edzi. Mantha amawombola. Mantha a tchalichi, kuopa abusa kumakupangitsa kuti usapezeke pamalo osayenera. Ngakhalenso mantha odulidwa mumpingo ukaphwanya chimo la chigololo. Izi zingamupangitse mzimayi kukhukupilira mwamuna mmodzi basi, osatenganso Edzi.*

witchcraft take advantage of the fragile health status of someone who has developed Aids. None of the clients from the ARV clinic claimed to have been bewitched.[130]

HIV Testing

Fear still prohibits most women from taking the initiative to know their HIV status. From the case study, not even a single woman has had her blood tested except seven women at the antenatal clinic. Even those from the Anglican Church are still afraid of the HIV test, and those newly married never bothered about testing before marriage. Culture does not force one to go for VCT; neither does it support someone who does. Religion and church at times encourage members to go for that. But this, as most women admitted, is seldom done. Although these women do not know their status, most said they find it difficult to initiate safe sex because they are not HIV positive. Many women think those that are HIV positive are the ones to use condoms.

> It is easier for someone who is HIV positive to use condoms because she fears spreading the virus. But for someone who is not, it is difficult. For how long will you use it?[131]

Surprisingly, when asked if it happens that they go for VCT and are diagnosed positive, will they be able to tell their partners? Most women said they cannot dare. It is impossible to do that for fear of being seen as promiscuous.

> He will ask where you got the virus. The best thing is to keep quiet and let him continue being suspicious of your losing weight. You can

---

[130] In other studies, equally limited as this one, there is a higher level of connections betweenHIV/Aids and witchcraft accusations.

[131] Int. Woman 17, 11.1.2005. *Wa edzi ndikwapafupi kugwiritsa ntchito kondomu. Nanga sakuopa kuti angapatsire mzake. Koma oti siukudziwa ndizovuta. Ugwiritsa mpaka liti?*

just be lying you are sick from stomachache. If you dare disclose it, he can send you back to your home to die there.[132]

Even unmarried women said that this is not an easy thing to do. Even when they may be found to be HIV positive, they said they cannot disclose it to their boyfriends for fear of losing the market. In order not to feel guilty, these women believe it is better not to go for an HIV test and continue their sexual life happily.

What kind of a man would want to have sex with a woman who is HIV positive? If you disclose your status, you will lose him automatically. He will never come back. To avoid such incidences and guilt of murdering an innocent person, it is better not to go for VCT.[133]

Most women believe a condom is a vital device for avoiding HIV/Aids. Many women said it is difficult to avoid HIV through abstinence and faithfulness, better use a condom, although it has its own hazards too.[134] Some of the women said that they heard that condoms are not reliable because they have 15 holes. Others said men deliberately pierce a condom with a needle.[135]

We have heard that when you are HIV positive, that is the end of your sexual life. You are not supposed to have sex with any man but only abstain. How can you live like that as if you are dead?[136]

---

[132] Int. Woman 31, 18.1.2005. *Aziti wakaitengera kuti, ndipovuta kunena kungokhala basi, angodabwira kuwonda, uzingoti cha m'mimba. Kungoyere-keza ndiye upakira wa kwanu, ukafere komweko.*

[133] Int. Woman 15, 10.1.2005. *Ndani mwamuna angalolere kugona ndi mkazi wa edzi. Kungomuuza ndiye sadzabweranso wamuluza ameneyo. Ndiye kuopa zonsezi chifukwa iwenso zizikupweleka mumtIma ukamaganiza kuti ukupha munthu osalakwa dala dala, ndi bwino osakayezetsa.*

[134] Int. Woman 8, 10.1.2005.

[135] I collected this information from Anglican women during focus group discussions at Mpira prayer house in 2005. *I expect that the level of information is better by now.

[136] Int. Group discussion 30.1.2005. *Tidamva kuti ukapezeka ndi kachilomboka ndiye kuti basi moyo wa m'banja wathera pomwepa. Akuti umafunika*

ARVs

Because all women from the case study do not know their HIV status, knowledge on ARVs is very little.[137] Many think ARV is a drug that cures HIV/Aids. The small percentage of women that seem to know that ARV is a drug that boosts the immune system, said they got this knowledge from antenatal clinics and sometimes from the radio. None heard it from the church. I was surprised that most women do not know there are ARVs within reach at St Luke's Hospital.

> We only have one type and this is a big challenge to those that may not fully respond to Triommune.[138]

At St Luke's, the percentage of women, since August 2004 when they started issuing the drug to January 2005, has reached 64% most of whom are unmarried.[139] Most clients from ARV clinic interviewed blamed their husbands to have sourced the virus for them. Many of

---

uzingokhala basi osagonananso ndi mwamuna. Ukhala bwanji munthu? Ngati wakufa hedee ilii.

[137] Even those clients from antenatal clinic at St Luke's do not have much knowledge of the drug. Clients from the ARV clinic responded reasonably well.

[138] Int. Laurens Boven, Acting Administrator, St Luke's, 19.1.2005. Dr Boven also cited following up of patients and inadequate supply of the drug as challenges. Because of this, not everyone who is HIV positive has access to ARV (From my discussion with women that are HIV positive in the same traditional area Malemia). As a representative of PLWAs in Zomba, I am in a position to talk and share experiences with those living with the virus. Of course, there are some not on ARV because of lack of knowledge, yet there are also others who are on the waiting list. Out of the 27 women from two groups, only two are on treatment. 17 are not on ARV due to lack of civic education and 8 have been told to wait. Triommune 30 is given to patients weighing less than 60 kg. Triommune 40 to those above 61 kg. *Treatment rules have changed since then and now there are more possibilities.

[139] Int. Laurens Boven, Acting Administrator, St Luke's, 19.1.2005. As to why most are unmarried, it is difficult to tell. Some women from Malemia commented that fear of their husbands bars them from taking an HIV test. Perhaps this could answer the question of why there are more unmarried women on ARV than those married.

these husbands died from TB. One woman talked about her experience as follows,

> I got married in 1989. I am a widow with three children. Vincent my first-born boy was born in 1992. Bright was born in 1996 and Ian in 2003. Ian was born at Lilongwe Central Hospital. My late husband was then working with Lever Brothers. My husband got ill immediately after Ian was born. It started with a mere cough, and then it was TB. He got worse and was wasting. He went for VCT in November 2003 at St Luke's Hospital where he was diagnosed HIV positive. I was advised to buy ARVs for my husband to survive but I could not afford. My husband died a month later. I am however grateful that his relatives did not grab the property after he died. I am still keeping all the *katundu* (property). Before he died, my husband gathered together his relatives and told them not to take anything from the house. I do not work so the property will assist me greatly. When in need, I can sell some of it. Ian was born prematurely at seven months old. He went for incubation for three weeks. Ian who is HIV positive is frequently ill with open bowels. At St Luke's, I have been told that the child cannot start ARV as he is still young.[140]

My husband was also diagnosed with TB. Of course, I do not blame him. I have forgiven him, but I am glad he knew before his death what killed him and how he got the HIV virus. I recall our relationship as follows.

> Dudley was the man I loved. From the very first day I saw him I knew he could keep me and care for me. Indeed, throughout the days he promised me love and I never doubted it. Our marriage took 10 months but in those few months, my life was different. He was my best friend and I enjoyed being called a wife. At last I had changed my status—now Mrs Maulana. In November 2001, he married me. I was to be his second wife. The first wife had died five years earlier,

---

[140] Int. Woman 45, 15.2.2005. This 32 year old widow, together with her children, stays with her parents. She started her ARVs from St Luke's in September 2004. Her major problem is food both for herself and the children. I saw the boy the time I was collecting my data. Despite his frequent illnesses, he looks charming and healthy. - *By now hospitals have special ARVs for children. And today, ARVs are free in district hospitals.

two years after they divorced. I never bothered to ask more about his sexual history, let alone the first marriage. There was no use. What mattered was that I was now married and my husband loved me. By January 2002, I was pregnant. I remember how much I danced when the doctor gave me the good news. It was going to be my first pregnancy at the age of 27. How glad my mother would be to hold a grandchild on her lap. I looked forward to it. Five months later, in May, the whole drama started. One morning, Dudley went to do some office work in Liwonde. Late in the evening when he came back, he started complaining of a headache. He was working with the Southern Region Water Board in Zomba. I thought it was an ordinary headache and gave him some painkillers. In the morning, he did not go to work. A week later, flu came with some itchy spots. Finally, it was a cough. I thought it was just another cough, possibly due to cold as we were in the winter season. After three weeks, we discovered it was more than the weather. He went for an X-ray at Zomba Central Hospital and Malamulo Adventist. At both places the result was negative. The cough continued, worse now. We went back to the hospital on 1st July with sputum. Indeed, he had TB. Immediately he started treatment, but he was already very weak. On 3rd September 2002, he closed his eyes before finishing his TB dose, dead.

few women, however, commented that they got what they deserved because of their own reckless lives. One woman who believes she got the virus from a bar spoke in this way.

I got it myself. I was mostly found in bars.[141]

Another woman says up to now she does not know how she got the virus. Her husband died in 1992 from TB. In 1997, after being sick for a long time, this woman went for an HIV test where she was diagnosed negative. In 2004, she got sick again.

It started with a simple cough. Later I was found with TB. I went for another HIV test at a VCT center in Balaka where I was diagnosed HIV positive. I could not believe it. From where did I get it? Even God in Heaven knows that the last man I slept with was my husband until today. Unless they made a mistake in 1997. Perhaps I got it

---

[141] Int. Woman 48, 1.2.2005. *Ine ndiye ndinazitengera. Kokhala kunali ku bala.*

from my job as a traditional birth attendant. But I still doubt it because I was always cautious.[142]

To most patients at St Luke's the drug is good in that it is easy to swallow and is not painful.[143] Most of those that are on treatment have improved tremendously.[144] On how they handle their sexual reproductive health, patients on ARV explained that they were advised by the service providers not to bear children for this is risky and also to abstain from casual sex. Emphasis on the use of condoms is given only to those that are married. One lady noted lack of clarity to unmarried people that are HIV positive on the use of condoms.

> We are told not to become pregnant for this is risky. They also tell us to abstain. Those that are married can use condoms. To those that are unmarried, condoms are not emphasized. Perhaps they
>
> think we are all married.[145]

Lack of highly nutritious food is the major challenge to those that are HIV positive in the area. Most of them are not only patients but also poor and uneducated and cannot afford to eat reasonably well. Apart from being uneducated, most of them are widows with a number of children to look after. Even those that are on ARV treatment seem to

---

[142] Int. Woman 46, 27.1.2005. The 45-year widow has three children. She admits that it has been a struggle to raise them single handedly. Two finished their secondary school last year. The last one is in form two. Woman 46 started ARVs in December 2004. Currently, she is taking both ARV and the TB treatment.

[143] Int. Woman 45, 5.3.2005. The tablet is taken twice a day, morning and evening.

[144] Despite some occasional side effects such as headaches, loss of appetite and body pains, most show a very positive development.

[145] Int. Woman 49, 10.3.2005. *Amatiwuza kuti kubelekanso uli ndi kachilombo ndi koopsa. Ndiponso tizidziletsa. Okha amene ali pa banja angathe kugwiritsa kondomu. Kwa amene sali pabanja sakambapo chili chonse. Mwina amawona ngati tonse tili pabanja.* From my contacts with PLWAs, I have noted some live a careless sexual life. It seems there is no one who tells them much.

on how they can handle their sexuality now that they are HIV positive.

struggle because of lack of nutritious food in their homes. At St Luke's Hospital, clients commented that sometimes they get Likuni flour to make porridge at their homes and BP5.[146]

Sexual Taboos and Initiation Teachings

Advice from Marriage Counsellors (anankungwi) concerning Sexual Life

During initiations and during traditional weddings, women are given some advice concerning life in the new home. A woman is told to respect her husband, cook for him, wash his clothes and cheer visitors. Sexual life is strongly emphasized. A woman is told that the biggest job in a family is sex. Even when she is sick or tired, a woman should not refuse her husband sex because once she does that, he would walk away to other women.[147] The women are also told never to cook for the family immediately after sex. Both the wife and the man must have a bath first.[148] Much emphasis is put on respecting the desires of their husbands. They are told to help the man during sex.

> It is not only the man that enjoys the pleasure of sex. Even you the lady feel the sweetness. So, make sure you do the job together, not just lying backwards.[149]

However, most women commented that nothing on reproductive health is said during the initiation. There is again no demonstration of

---

[146] Int. Woman 46, 10.3.2005. BP 5 is a type of nutrient food in form of biscuits. Because of inadequate supply from the donor, this is not always in stock and when it comes it is often in small quantities.

[147] Int. Woman 21, 12.1.2005.

[148] Int. Woman 20, 12.1.2005.

[149] Int. Woman 10, 10.1.2005. *Kukoma sikusankha. Mumamva nonse. Ndiye kumagwilira limodzi ntchito osati kumangogona gada! heheeee* This lady commented that sometimes men tend to leave their wives and seek assistance from some girlfriends because of the way their wives behave in bed. They just lie on their back without doing anything waiting for the man to do the job alone.

how a woman should handle her man in bed.[150] Most women said perhaps this is taken for granted as everyone knows how to do it while there may be those that do not know anything at all. Some women again said although they are sometimes taught the sexual dance during *chinamwali*, this is however difficult to remember after years have gone by when you grow up. A small girl can easily shake her hips. This is not always simple and possible when you get older. A woman is also told not to be afraid to have sex with a man because age does not matter.[151] Below are some of the songs sung during *chinamwali* of *litiwo* and *liputu*.[152]

Song 5

One: Chinamwali chalero	One: Today's initiation
All: Iyaiyaiyaiya	All: Iyaiyaiyaiya
One: Chandipatsa mavuto.	One: It has given me trouble.
All: Iyaiyaiyaiya	All: Iyaiyaiyaiya
One: Mabvuto akuchipinda	One: Troubles in the bedroom
All: Iyaiyaiyaiya	All: Iyaiyaiyaiya
All: Dendekudendeku	All: Dendekudendeku
Dendekudendeku wa wa!	Dendekudendeku wa wa![153]

Song 6

One: Kanthuko, kanthuko,	One: That thing, that thing,
All: Kali mchiunomu.	All: It is around the waist.
One: Kanthuko, kanthuko	One: That thing, that thing
All: Kali mchiunomu.	All: It is around the waist.
One: Kayendayenda kayendayenda	One: It is moving about

---

[150] Int. Woman 2, 8.1.2005.

[151] Int. Woman 21, 12.1.2005. The text they use to refer to this is *Seveni tani galimoto yolimba*. (Seven tons is a strong car). The seven-ton car symbolizes the vagina that can accommodate both small and big penis. It is regarded as strong.

[152] *Litiwo* takes place at home, while *chiputu*, a girls' initiation, takes place in the bush.

[153] Meaning of the song is to get the woman ready for the man to make love to her. The song was sung with styles of shaking the hips. During my study, I was happy to see some women dancing to the tune beautifully.

All: Pachabe amangwetu,
kali lendelendee

All: In vain, friends, it is just hanging.[154]

Song 7

One: Ndiuzeni,
All: Ndiuzeni nyini yankhuku

One: Tell me
All: Tell me the vagina of the chicken

One: Ee eya eya eee.

All: Ee eya eya eee.[155]

Song 8

One: Kadam'manja, Kadam'manja,

One: Kadam'manja, Kadam'manja,

All: dedede
One: Dzulo, lero,
wam'menya mayi wako,
All; dedede,
One: Wamuyesa Kadam'manja.
All: dedede.

All: dedede
One: Yesterday, today,
you beat your mother,
All: dedede,
One: As if she is Kadam'manja
All: dedede.[156]

---

[154] The meaning of the song is the same as above. "Kali lende lende" is the penis that is just hanging waiting to go somewhere. *Amangwetu* is a Yao word like the Nyanja *Anzanga* (friends).

[155] This song was sung during *Chinamwali* to emphasize *zokoka*. This was to tell the initiates that it is not only women who have a vagina, chicken also have one. Rachel Fiedler comments that the chicken vagina is also used to teach the initiates "Kuthona-kukoka" - to lengthen the labia (Rachel NyaGondwe Fiedler, *Coming of Age. A Christianized Initiation among Women in Southern* Malawi, Zomba: Kachere, 2005, p. 34 and 69).

[156] The song depicts respect to the elder. During *chinamwali*, girls are also taught to respect their parents and other elder people. Kadam'manja has no meaning. It was like a name of a person who does not respect her mother and beats her daily. The literal meaning is someone with dirty hands. This song also encourages the girls to assist their mothers in domestic work and not to take her as a slave (with dirty hands). See Rachel NyaGondwe Fiedler, *Coming of Age. A Christianized Initiation among Women in Southern Malawi*, Zomba: Kachere, 2005, p. 63 for a similar negative connotation of the name Kadam'manja.

Cultural Beliefs and Customs

Each culture has its own customs and beliefs unique to its people or being shared with others. Women from Malemia explain the following beliefs that are in their area. Some cultural practices that seem to promote HIV/Aids are not available in this area. These include *fisi*, *kuchotsa fumbi* and no sex after menopause. All women said they just hear about these customs but they are not practised in their area. None of the widows reported to have undergone the practice of *kuchotsa fumbi* after the death of her husband.[157]

---

[157] Even myself, I did not undergo this tradition when my husband died. But I still recall seven months later, a neighbour in the location I was residing, someone I considered a *mother* (and indeed do so even today) told me of a certain *mwambo* that made me shed tears afterwards. She called me one day, sat me down and said she loved me. Because of such affection, she decided to clear her thoughts. I was confused but she kept on talking. "Pakufunika mupeze mwamuna wina achotse zoipazo. Ndichikonditu sichoncho amayi. Kupanda kuchotsa zimenezo simudzabelekanso. Inetu ndimakukondani ngati mwana wanga. Sindimafuna kuti mudzakhumate osabeleka. Mukanali mtsikana. Mwandimva...." (You need to find a man to clear the filth. What I am saying here is out of love. If that is not removed, you will never bear children again. I love you as my daughter and I would not be happy to see you one day gloomy and childless. You are still young, go you hear this...). This remark came as another nightmare in my life, indeed a dilemma. Should I remain childless forever because of something I could have avoided, how I wish I could nurse an infant of my own one day or should I just go out in the streets looking for a man to sleep with, and do I know what killed my husband. What if I am HIV positive? This was a difficult moral issue to decide. I told my friends Jacqueline Chazema and Mirriam Kumwenda who reminded me to cast my burden unto God. They assured me that if God had planned that I have children, I would have them regardless of the tradition. Mirriam dedicated herself through prayers and indeed healed my mind. This is indeed how HIV is spread. If I had obliged to the woman's wish, I would have infected an innocent man who could have infected his wife or his sexual partner who could again take it to their sexual partners and so on and on. It is a chain (see appendix 3). Thank God for giving me the courage to resist that practice. I could have been feeling guilty now. But I don't blame her. In fact I love her very much and still regard her as a *mother*. It's a

We do not have that tradition here. I think one's marriage could break with that practice. I had my menopause at the age of 45, now I am 62. You mean all these years between, we could just have been keeping each other as children? The man cannot allow that. Even I, as a woman, cannot manage to look at my husband as if he were a tree [158]

Women believe if such practice is evident in some areas, it is useless and impossible. To these women, this kind of tradition means deliberately selling your husband to other women.

Should a man be keeping you as if you are a child? For sure he would go out looking for a girlfriend because you are *dead*. A man does not grow old. A woman is different in such that she loses her sexual desire after giving birth.[159]

Most women from the sample said they adhere to the cultural beliefs available in their area. To most women, it is their husbands that fail to follow most practices. Ignoring cultural taboos, to most women, is what has contributed to HIV/Aids. For instance, neglect of the sexual practice of abstinence (*mwambo wa kudikha*) has made HIV/Aids increase. In the past, people were afraid to break any law or belief for fear of *mdulo*. At times, a lawbreaker could be taken to the traditional court for punishment. Women from the sample commented that today *mdulo*

---

pity she would not know that I never carried out her desire. Neither do I wish to let her know. It is no use.

[158] Int. Woman 7, 7.5.2005 *Kulibe mwambo umenewo kuno. Ndiye mpaka banja litathatu. Ine ndinasiya kusamba ndili ndi zaka 45. Pano ndili 62, ndiye mukundiuza kuti zaka zonsezi, tachotserani ndi zingati, tizingosungana m'nyumbamu ngati mwana. Ndiye banjalo likhalapo. Mpaka litatha, mwamunayo angalore zopusazo. Ndiponso ngakhale ine mkazi, tisamangoti amuna okha, sindingakwanitse kumangomuyang'ana mwamuna wanga ngati ndi mtengo.*

[159] Int. Woman 10, 30.4.2005. Should a man be keeping you as if you are a child? For sure he would go out looking for a girlfriend because you are *dead*. A man does not grow old. A woman is different in such that she loses her sexual desire after giving birth. *Mwamunayo azingokulera ngati mwana wake? Ndiye apita kuchibwenzi. Nanga iwe siwafa. Mwamuna sathelapo ngakhale atakalamba. Mkazi amasiyana ndi mwamuna, chilakolako chimatha msanga akabeleka.*

66

taboos are no longer stressed. As a result, most people are not afraid to break them

Pregnancy related taboos

In Malemia, women are required to observe some customs when pregnant. A pregnant mother is expected to take much care during pregnancy. Just like the Tumbuka, the Yao believe that the life of a child begins with pregnancy. One such care is through proper management of her sexual life. When a woman has conceived, couples continue with sexual intercourse until the pregnancy is seven months old. The foetus inside the mother's belly needs food to grow. Some of this food is taken from the father's semen. This is for the well-being and health of the baby. Like in the Tumbuka tradition, the man's sperm is believed to feed the baby as it develops.

> Sexual intercourse during this time is necessary as it nourishes the child. Without this, the baby is born very weak and with very low birth weight. In some cases, the woman may even have a stillbirth.[160]

In the last two months of the pregnancy, sexual intercourse is put on hold. The pregnant mother is not supposed to have sex, a practice of abstinence known as *mipingu*. This was not only to avoid *mdulo* or *tsempho*,[161] but it is believed that a child born with sperms covering its body will be very weak and might eventually die.[162] A few women from my sample commented that midwives shout at them if they see any semen during delivery, as they get disgusted.[163] Birth attendants strongly advise expectant mothers not to have sex a few days before

---

[160] Ibid. p. 126. Sexual intercourse is compared to the fertilizer a maize plant needs at different stages in order to grow well.

[161] This was believed to occur to those that breach cultural beliefs e.g. eating relish salted by a menstruating woman. During certain periods, women are considered cold. Therefore to have sex with a man who is hot could have dire consequences. Even newborn babies could be victims of *tsempho*.

[162] The creamy substance that covers the body of the baby is *vernix caseosa*, which protects the foetus from amniotic fluid and from friction against itself.

[163] Int. Woman 8, 11.1.2005.

delivery. Sexual abstinence during this time is also seen as important to prevent harm to the foetus. It is perceived that the man's penis may pierce the child's fontanel. Abstinence should therefore take place for fear of damaging the fontanel (*liwombo*).

> When the power of the man is so intense, his penis can knock the head of the baby, damaging the fontanel.[164]

From my study, 45 women had at least one pregnancy in their lifetime. Out of these, only three women abstained completely in their last months until they delivered. The rest said that at times they could have sex when the desire for it was too intense.[165]

In Malemia, pregnant mothers go through the ritual of *litiwo*. During one's first pregnancy, a woman is supposed to be initiated. The *litiwo* is a dance that takes place in the open ground right at the woman's home.[166]

Song 9

Kuwotcha, akukanga,	To feel hot, she is failing,
Kutanda unya manyi mwana.	You produce stool before the child comes out.
Mwana asanatuluke,	Before the child comes out
Uyamba kusanza	You start vomiting
Mwana asanatuluke.	Before the child comes out.[167]

---

[164] Int. Woman 10, 10.1.2005. *Mphamvu ya mwamuna ikakula chiwalo chake chingathe kugunda mutu wa mwana, kuwononga liwombo.* This woman, who strongly claims that there is no HIV/Aids but Kanyera, says men have killed themselves today because of failure to keep "mipingu" (*mwambo*). In the past, she says, there was a medicine for *kanyera* from traditional healers, but today such medicine is no longer there. Apart from *liwombo* and *kanyera*, another illness of a child is *likango*. *Likango* (Herpes) is a nasty illness that may at times kill even the parents if not treated on time.

[165] During such periods, the woman is expected to sleep with the husband sideways and not lying on her back.

[166] Int. Women 10, 10.1.2005.

[167] Ibid.

Song 10

Chitetete,	Nothing is done,
Zuwali, zuwali, kukalowa.	This sun, this sun, to go and set,
Zuwa ndi kutuluka.	The sun comes out.[168]

The tradition of *litiwo* is not a must but it is a necessity. Those who do not want to be initiated for their own reasons are not forced to do so. However, from my sample, all women went through this during their first pregnancy. One woman who was initiated in 2001 spoke of her experience as follows.

> My mother went through *litiwo*. During my first pregnancy, she called some counsellors for me. She said I should be initiated too because she also went through the same. They do it on the open ground. Only those that have been initiated are allowed to attend the ceremony. Those who have not are not permitted. Many people came to watch it. There were four counsellors (*anankungwi*). It is funny. They dance (see song below) and counsel you when you are putting on only a skirt.[169]

One: Elo elo	One: Elo elo
All: Elo elo	All: Elo elo
One: Wanyole, wanyole	One: Shaving, shaving
All: Wanyole, wanyole	All: Shaving, shaving
One: Malezasi fayifi atchoka	One: Five razor blades have broken
All: Watoladyi akulukutile.	All: Take another one to finish.[170]

---

[168] Ibid.

[169] Int. Woman 22, 17.1.2005. *Ine mayi anga anavinidwa litiwo. Ndiye ine ndili ndi mimba yanga yoyamba, anandiitanira anankungwi. Anati ndi vinidwenso poti iwo anavididwa. Amavinira pabwalo. Amene amawalora kuti adzawonere ndi okhaokhawo amene anavinidwa litiwo. Osavinidwa samamulora. Kunabwera anthu ambiri odzawonera. Anankungwi analipo folo. Zimasangalatsa. Amavina ndi kumakulangiza utavala siketi yokha.*

[170] The song (in Yao) depicts the importance of frequent shaving of one's private parts.

Sexual faithfulness is much stressed during *litiwo* initiation. The pouring of castor oil on the forehead of the pregnant mother is one essence of *litiwo* that is given the name of *chipendo*.[171] The oil is supposed to run vertically straight across her navel towards her vagina if she was faithful at the conception of the pregnancy.[172] It is also believed that if there is a woman who committed adultery with the husband of this woman, during the anointing time, the woman would lose her pregnancy at the same time.[173] The ritual of *chipendo* is primarily done to ensure faithfulness in marriage.

Delivery taboos

Immediately after delivery, a woman is not supposed to cook for the family for some time. These periods vary but most said at least one month. A woman is also required to follow hygiene and bath at least three times a day.[174] Sexual abstinence is again to be followed for a period of at least 8 months.[175] If, however, it was a stillbirth delivery, the parents should abstain for 4 months.[176] In the past elderly women said they followed this practice and no sex took place until the baby was 8 months old. The reason was to avoid *mdulo*. When a couple fails to adhere to sexual regulations during this time, it is believed that the newborn child may suffer from *tsempho* and may die. This kind of sexual abstinence was another way of family planning. A woman is strictly instructed not to have sex with her husband for the sake of the baby.

Likambako

Immediately when the baby is born, it is bathed in water containing herbs made from *likambako*. *Likambako* is a ritual to protect the

---

[171] Rachel NyaGondwe Banda, *Women of Bible and Culture. Baptist Convention Women in Southern Malawi*, Zomba: Kachere, 2005, p. 27.

[172] Ibid.

[173] Ibid.

[174] Int. Woman 27, 13.1.2005.

[175] Int. Woman 11, 20.1.2005.

[176] Int. Woman 4, 7.1.2005.

newborn baby. A string is put around the waist and neck of the baby. Today's women often refuse this because they say *mzachikunja* (it is non-Christian) and *zachimidzi* (traditional).[177] This is a traditional medicine given to the baby to avoid *tsempho*. *Likambako* was not free. It was bought from a traditional healer. After 8 months, the baby was again given some *likambako*. After bathing it, the couple was now ready to resume sexual life.[178]

Kanyera

This was a very common disease in the past; it was associated with *mdulo*. To avoid it, most people adhered to cultural practices. The signs of *kanyera* include lean fingers, being skinny, pain below the man's navel, feeling of coldness and continuous desire for fire.[179] In those days, there was traditional medicine for such a disease and people could be cured. Today such medicine is no longer there. A few women from my sample strongly argued that there is no such a disease as HIV/Aids but *kanyera*. It is difficult for people in rural areas to distinguish patients of *kanyera* from those of HIV/Aids because of similarities in symptoms.[180] One woman commented that men are killing themselves for failure to follow *mwambo wa kudikha* (sexual abstinence).[181]

---

[177] Int. Woman 3, 9.1.2005.

[178] Int. Woman 6, 9.1.2005.

[179] Int. Woman 10, 10.1.2005.

[180] In some areas, *kanyera* is known as *chinyera*. Cf. Rachel NyaGondwe Fiedler, *Coming of Age. A Christianized Initiation among Women in Southern* Malawi, Zomba: Kachere, 2005, p. 29. The author comments that *chinyera* is perceived to be curable through traditional herbs. She further argues that there is need to educate women on the Christian perspective on menstrual blood and the realities of HIV/Aids in their communities. She believes that this would liberate women to have sexual relations during menstruation if they so desire. She observes that some women know that having sexual intercourse during such a period is advantageous when some women desire to have sex. Besides, it is a time when one is unable to conceive and therefore good for those using natural methods of birth control.

[181] Int. Woman 10, 10.1.2005.

Menstruation related taboos

This practice is also still there in Malemia. All women from the sample said they abide by this tradition. They also do this for hygienic reasons. Other beliefs like not adding salt while menstruating are not practised in this area. In this area, it is also sometimes emphasized that during such periods a woman should not share drinking water with her husband. All this is to avoid *tsempho* or *mdulo.* Touching menstrual blood could lead to dire consequences such as *kanyera.* All women say, the moment they finish menstruating, they are free to indulge in sex. When a woman is menstruating, she is perceived as unclean.[182]

> A man can die. It is the same with sleeping with a man after stillbirth. A man dies. It just needs proper care. You know it yourself as the woman when you are through with your menstruating. Medication is there. If you seek it quickly from the traditional healer, there is a chance of survival. But most men hide it because of shame and they continue sick. By the time, they reveal it to people it is already too late.[183]

One woman commented that once it happened to her by accident. She thought she had finished menstruating and had sexual intercourse with her husband. However, the husband never got sick 'as was the case in the past.'[184]

Lengthening of the labia minora (zokoka)

Apart from the sexual dance taught during *chinamwali,* another way of satisfying a man in bed is elongation of the labia. It was strongly em-

---

[182] Compare Leviticus 15 about ritual uncleanliness of menstruating women. During those biblical times, sexual intercourse with such women was forbidden.

[183] Int. Woman 22, 3.6.2005. *Mwamuna angathe kumwalira. Chimodzimodzi kugona ndi mwamuna utachita chitayo. Mwamuna amafa. Zimafunika kusamala. Umadziwa wekha kuti wamaliza kusamba. Mankhwala koma alipo. Ukafulumira kupita kwa a sing'anga amachira. Koma ena amabisa, osanene akuti manyazi ndi kumangodwala. Mmene azidzanena kwa anthu mochedwa. Kusamba* is a common Chichewa term for menstruation. Other words include *kumwezi* (to be on the moon).

[184] Int. Woman 32, 25.1.2005.

phasized in the past. From my study, those that have *zokoka*, are less in number than those without. Most of those women are in the late 30s and above. This group of women believes *zokoka* is an important concept and strengthens family life. These women feel it is not surprising that some men have extramarital affairs because of absence of *zokoka* from their wives.

> *Makwelero* is a ladder. *Zokoka* is more like decorations. (A woman should not be like a baby, plain (private parts) without ladders.)[185]

Most women say *zokoka* is very important in sexual life, mainly to arouse the man in bed, although some young women today tend to ignore that and do not have them.

> The man's part (penis) wakes up quickly when he is playing with the labia.[186]

The lengthening of the labia minora is not only emphasized in traditional initiations but also by the church. Molly Longwe comments on the importance of *zokoka* in the church. During *chilangizo,* the girls were asked to open their legs and show the counsellors if they were pulling their labia minora.[187] *Zokoka* strengthens the sexual life of the couple and binds the marriage. A few women commented that absence of *zokoka* could lead to divorce.

---

[185] Int. woman 11, 20.1.2005. *Mkazi asamakhale ngati mwana ali mbee opanda makwelero.*

[186] Int. Woman 6, 9.1.2005. *Chiwalo cha mwamuna chimadzuka msanga mwamuna akamaseweretsa zokoka.* Accordingly, the woman has the freedom to be touching the man's genitals. In so doing, it is very easy for both of them to get aroused easily.

[187] See Molly Longwe, "From Chinamwali to Chilangizo: The Christianization of Pre-Christian Chewa Initiation Rites in the Baptist Convention of Malawi", MTh, University of Natal, Pietermaritzburg, 2003, pp. 85ff. Published as: Molly Longwe, *Growing Up. A Chewa Girls' Initiation*, Zomba: Kachere, 2006.

Marriages break. Men from Ntcheu or Lilongwe, when they marry here and find out that the wife does not have them, the marriage breaks.[188]

Another woman commented that women whose marriages are about to break come to seek medicine from her on *zokoka*. Such women come from different areas in Zomba and some even from Mangochi and Blantyre.[189]

Conclusion

This chapter has described the experiences of women in sexual and reproductive health. It can be concluded that sexual life, to most women in Malemia, whether married or unmarried, is a prerequisite. Women play a small role on issues concerning their sexual and reproductive life. The woman has a limited place in decision-making concerning the couple's sexual and reproductive lives. Men seem to dominate in all issues of sexual and reproductive health in the homes. They are in charge of sexual intercourse. Culture does not permit a woman to ask for sex from her partner. It is a taboo. The study also found out that nakedness seems not to be appreciated in most homes. Most couples are ashamed to dress and undress in front of each other.

---

[188] Int. Woman 11, 20.1.2005. *Mabanja amatha. Azibambo aku Ntcheu, kaya uku ku Lilongwe akakwatiwa kuno ndi kupeza kuti mkazi alibe, limatha banja.* Compare J.C. Chakanza, "The Unfinished Agenda: Puberty Rites and the Response of the Roman Catholic Church in Southern Malawi", in *Religion in Malawi*, no. 5, 1995, p. 4. Chakanza shows that there is a perception that lack of elongation of labia minora encourages divorce.

[189] Int. Woman 10, 10.1.2005. "To lengthen the labia minora, one just needs to mix some traditional herbs with castor oil. All my fellow ladies who would want to meet this woman consult me and I will give you directions."

A Woman's Cry

Sister,
If you happen to meet him
Tell him that in matrimony
Hands are for caressing the wife's body
And fondling her breasts
Not a sjambok
For whipping her body
or slapping her face.

Sister, sister
If you see the man
Forget not to remind him
That a man's chest in bed
Is the woman's pillow
Where she can pour her tears
In times of sorrow as well as joy
Not hardboard for manifesting his temper.

Sister, sister, please
If by chance you meet your brother-in-law
Whisper in his ears that in marriage lips are for kissing
And producing sweet nonsense
Thereby giving pleasure to each other
Not for kissing a calabash of beer
producing words fit for the bin thereafter.

Sister, sister, please, sister,
If you encounter the man I married
Remember to say to him that his eyes
Are there to admire his wife
The shape of her body
The beauty of her face
And the art of her hands
Not to lust after teenage girls.

Sister, sister, please, sister, Abiti Moya,
If you meet CHEJAFARI, my husband,
Deliver to him this message:

Money in the home should be there
To maintain wife and young ones
Not to purchase risky pleasures
Which he can have free and safe
From me, his wife, Abiti Daniel.

Cecilia Hasha

Chapter 3: The Anglican Church and Women's Sexuality

It is obvious that life is a challenge to women, especially today in the context of HIV/Aids. A careless sexual and reproductive life can have dire consequences. Similarly, with HIV/Aids, child birth is a challenge, especially in making sure that every pregnancy is wanted and that the delivery itself and the coming baby are safe and free from the virus. How the Anglican Church has responded to such moral issues of women's sexuality is the focus of this chapter.

Biblical Principles and Teachings on Women's Sexuality

For Christians, the Bible teaches fundamental truths about human behaviour.[190] Christianity teaches that sex is a divine gift. Therefore, it demands responsibility, commitment and total love. Sex is the most beautiful expression of a deep loving and life-long relationship between two people. It is a great blessing. Helmut Thielicke believes that sexuality is a dimension of human existence itself, and thus a mystery just as man is.[191] Marriage is an order of creation grounded in the primeval relationship of the sexes and a constituent part of the created things.[192] It is a divine institution, willed and protected by God himself. This is the primary reason why this order of creation must be upheld.

> Submit to one another out of reverence for Christ. Wives should submit to their husbands as to the Lord. Now as the Church submits to Christ, so also wives should submit to their husbands in everything. Husbands love your wives, just as Christ loved the church and gave himself up for her. Husbands ought to love their

---

[190] Joe Jenkins notes that the church finds itself in the situation where its teachings often seem old-fashioned and out of place in a world where sexual ethics are fast changing. See Joe Jenkins, *Contemporary Moral Issues*, Oxford: Heinemann, 1997, p. 52.

[191] Helmut Thielicke, *The Ethics of Sex*, New York: Harper and Row, 1964, p. 64. The author comments that a mystery is always a sign that something vulnerable is to be protected.

[192] Ibid., p. 104.

wives as their own bodies. He who loves his wife loves himself. After all, no one ever hated his own body, but feeds and cares for it, just as Christ does the church.[193]

Another purpose of marriage is to re-produce. The great cosmic purpose of sex is the survival of our species.[194] Children are a gift of God so that the human race can survive. However, Helmut Thielicke considers the procreation of children as only a partial component of marriage subsumed under, and derived from its main purpose namely, the mutual interior formation of husband and wife.[195] The most important thing in a Christian marriage is love between the spouses.[196]

On Women's Role

In the beginning, God created woman and man equal as stated in Genesis 1 and 2.[197] God's original will is equality. Unlike the Israelite history that purely deals with the story of Abraham and Sarah plus their families, the story of creation is a story with a message to the entire humanity.[198] It is not history per se, neither is it an ordinary story. The story of creation is valid for all of us and for all times, written so that we understand how God wants us to live.[199] It is a tool which helps us to

---

[193] Ephesians 5:21-25, 29 NIV. Paul emphasizes that submission should be done out of reverence for Christ. A man has to sacrifice for his wife's life as Christ sacrificed for the Church. The text gives no permission to the man to mistreat his wife but speaks of mutual submission and the man's sacrifice.

[194] Eric Berne, *Sex in Human Loving*, Harmondsworth: Penguin, 1973, p. 49.

[195] Helmut Thielicke, *The Ethics of Sex*, p. 204.

[196] Kristina Baker and Honor Ward, *Aids, Sex and Family Planning*, Achimota: Africa Christian Press, 1989, p. 22.

[197] Genesis 1:27 says: "So God created man in his own image, in the image of God he created him; male and female he created them" (NIV). In *Buku Loyera*, man is translated *munthu* with no distinction as to whether the *munthu* is male or female.

[198] Janet Kholowa and Klaus Fiedler, *In the Beginning God Created them Equal*, Blantyre: CLAIM-Kachere, 2003, p. 10.

[199] Ibid., p. 11.

understand God's will and to show us where we are wrong.[200] The same equality was emphasized when Adam saw that the woman God had created was exactly like him. She was a help fit for him: "This is now bone of my bones and flesh of my flesh. She shall be called a woman, for she was taken out of man."[201]

God blessed them and said to them, "Be fruitful and increase in number, fill the earth and subdue it. Rule over the fish of the sea and the birds of the air and over every living creature that moves on the ground."[202]

The other misunderstanding comes from Paul's writings. For instance, in his letter to the Ephesians, Paul talks of a woman's submission to her husband. Yet this kind of submission is out of reverence for Christ and nothing else,[203] and it is mutual.[204] On the same, another misconception comes when interpreting 1 Corinthians 7 which talks about marriage as a way of avoiding immorality. Paul indeed argues that marriage is appropriate for morality. However, to believe that this is the idea of marriage is another misconception. Avoiding immorality is just a side effect and not the purpose of marriage.[205]

---

[200] Ibid., p. 12.

[201] Genesis 2:23 NIV.

[202] Genesis 1:28 NIV.

[203] The English word submit is translated "obey" in Buku Lopatulika. "*Komatu monga Eklesia amvera Kristu, koteronso akazi amvere amuna ao m'zinthu zonse*" (Ephesians 5:24).

[204] Ephesians 5:21.

[205] The Book of Common Prayer of 1559 depicts avoiding fornication as one argument for marriage. It reads: "Secondly, it was ordained for remedy agaynste sinne and to avoide fornication, that suche persones as have not the gifte of continencie might marry, and kepe temeselves undefiled members of Christes body." See *The Book of Common Prayer – 1559: The Fourme of Soleminizacion of Matrimonye*, http://justus.anglican.org/resources/bcp/ 1559/Marriage_1559.htm, p. 1, 23.11.2005. This line of reasoning is not presented in *The Alternative Service Book 1980*, which is the English language prayer book Anglicans in the Upper Shire diocese use. See, *The Alternative Service Book 1980*, Cambridge: Cambridge University Press, 1980, p. 288.

God did not create another *adam*, but *isha* who was different from *adam*, hence the differences in nouns. Adam contributed to the creation of gender differentiation for in his exclamation of joy of finding someone like himself, Adam calls this being *isha*, who was obviously different from *adam* or *ish*.[206]

Apart from being created, biblically, gender differentiation was also recognized. God accepted it in his plan that the two genders are different. In Genesis 3, after the fall of humankind, God uses gender terms of woman and man, wife and husband in his recognition of gender. Nevertheless, despite this distinction, there is absolutely no clue that dictates female marginalization.

Eve's life revolves around pain in child birth, sexual passion for her husband and her humiliating subservience to her husband. Her partner becomes her master. Sexuality is now distorted to become the domination of one partner over the other.[207]

In the gospel of Mathew, one of the teachers of the law wanted to trick Jesus on the issue of divorce, whether it is lawful for a man to divorce his wife for each and every reason.[208] In his answer, Jesus quoted

---

[206] Hilary Mijoga, "Gender Differentiation in the Bible: Created and Recognized" in *Journal of Humanities*, no. 13, UNIMA, 1999, p. 88. The author comments that in Genesis 1 and 2, gender differentiation does not depict any marginalization of the female gender. After the creation of the woman, man (*munthu*) was no longer alone but in duality. Mijoga adds that it is in this dependence on the other that his creatureliness consists (p. 89).

[207] Ibid., p. 94. The author comments that after this incident, Adam did not accuse his wife for the sin but that after realizing their nakedness, they sewed fig leaves together.

[208] See Mathew 19:3. The teachers of the law differed on divorce. There was Shammai who taught that a man may divorce his wife for a serious reason, that is, marital infidelity. On the other hand Hillel believed that a man had the power to divorce his wife for any reason, even for him not liking her any more. Their teachings were both based on the Law of Moses, in particular the book of Deuteronomy. "If a man marries a woman who becomes displeasing to him because he finds something indecent about her, and he writes her a certificate of divorce, gives it to her and sends her from his house" (Deut 24:1 NIV). For

neither Deuteronomy nor the Law of Moses, but rather referred to Genesis and the story of creation.[209] Besides, he also jumped Genesis 3:16. By referring to Genesis, Jesus wanted to show that people should not look for an answer in the Law of Moses, but in what God said in the beginning (and for all times).[210]

Marriage in the Anglican Sense

The Church of England views marriage as "a gift of God, blessed by Christ and a symbol of Christ's relationship with the Church."[211] The Anglican Church in the Upper Shire Diocese, like most Christian churches, views marriage as a permanent union.[212] Besides, Anglicans believe in the marriage vow made at one's wedding ceremony, which ends with the words "till death do us part".[213]

> The commitment is until death, whether you will be bored with each other along the way, whether one is promiscuous and seems to threaten one's life, that is not an issue.[214]

According to the Anglican Church, only a monogamous marriage is permissible. Yet in public opinion, polygamy is still a proper marriage and popularly supported. Both monogamy and polygamy from the

---

details see Janet Kholowa and Klaus Fiedler, *In the Beginning God Created them Equal*, Blantyre: CLAIM-Kachere, 2000, p. 13.

[209] Ibid., p. 13.

[210] Ibid.

[211] Ibid.

[212] I attended a wedding officiated by Fr Francis Chipala at Likwenu parish in Chilema on 5th June 2004. The whole church was amidst ululations as Winnie smiled and spoke confidently making a covenant with Opes, "I, Winnie, do solemnly swear to take thee, Opes, to have and to hold, from this day forward, for better for worse, for richer for poorer, in sickness and in health, till death do us part."

[213] See Edward Stevens, *Making Moral Decisions*, New York: Paulist Press, 1969, p. 91.

[214] Ibid. Stevens considers this view of marriage as problematic.

stand point of man in society are valid forms of marriage.[215] Polygamy seemed to be there in the biblical times. However, by Christian standards and in terms of social development, monogamy is the order of the future.[216] It is the accepted order in wider parts of the OT and completely so in the New Testament.[217]

According to the clergy, through the gift of sex, God brings another gift, the children and desires that they be brought up in accordance with God's will, to his praise and glory.[218] Although the objective of married life is not simply to bear children, they, however, play a vital role in almost all families. Children are the outcome of the union of a woman and a man. One priest called this a continuation of God's work in creation.[219]

Sexuality in the Anglican Sense

Anglicans believe that man and woman are equal partners and helpers (*athandizi*).[220] For any job to be done there is need for someone on equal footing so that you move together.[221] In the understanding of the Church, to submit is not to be ruled but to do things together.[222] As such, there is need for communication and understanding between couples in a family. At the same time, this equality gives security to the other. The clergy believes that even when it is commonly asserted that the man is the head of the family, in reality one cannot survive with the head alone.

---

[215] Hans Häselbarth, *Christian Ethics in the African Context*, Ibadan: Daystar, 1976, p. 72.

[216] Ibid.

[217] For a discussion of polygamy and the church see: Moses Mlenga, *Polygamy in Northern Malawi. A Christian Perspective*, Mzuzu: Mzuni Press, 2016.

[218] Int. Fr. Francis Chipala, Likwenu parish priest, Liwonde, 28.1.2005.

[219] Ibid.

[220] Int. Fr Martin Mgeni, Mangochi parish priest, Zomba, 19.7.2005.

[221] Ibid.

[222] Ibid.

In marriage seminars, what we advise is how they can maintain their marriage. The problem in most families is lack of satisfaction. How do you get the satisfaction? Through understanding one another. Learn from one another. If you do not understand or are not open with one another, for example, at how you do the budgeting in your home, things cannot work. You cannot do it wholesale.[223]

To members of the clergy, sexual intercourse acts as a catalyst of love between the two.[224] It is like an entertainment in most homes. Members of the clergy believe marriage was constituted to ensure sexual union. One member spoke as follows.

A man cannot live alone otherwise life could be boring. A woman is there to fill up that loneliness. God teaches that love is the fulfillment of the law. One of Jesus Christ's teachings was to summarize that all the laws are bound in one golden law of love. In marriage, the church tries to put this into practice. The wedlock consists of two different people brought in from different backgrounds and beliefs. Man and woman tend to learn from one another. This involves self-denial, perseverance, kindness, offering one another the best things you think will please the other partner. This must be true love without condition.[225]

To most women from the study, their presence in the home matters a lot. Women believe life becomes a complete unit with a woman. Without them, life is like an empty nest. Accordingly, a home needs a woman to make it complete.

---

[223] Int. Fr. Martin Mgeni, Zomba, 19.7.2005.

[224] Whereas Christians believe that sex outside marriage is wrong mainly because Jesus said so. Joe Jenkins further points out that sexual intercourse between a couple who love one another and intend to create a life together is morally acceptable. See Joe Jenkins, *Contemporary Moral Issues*, Oxford: Heinemann, 1997, p. 35.

[225] Int. Brightone Malasa, Bishop's chaplain, Malosa, 2.3.2005. Fr. Brighton Malasa is now the sitting Bishop of the Upper Shire Diocese.

> Perhaps girls, these recent marriages. We never got any counselling concerning sexual life.[226]

Findings from the study reveal some decrease of church weddings in the Anglican Church. Most Anglican women, just as the clergy observed, do not undergo church weddings (*ukwati woyera*). Most marriages in the church today are blessed marriages (*ukwati wodalitsa*). A wedding in the Anglican Church is an achievement on the way and not the beginning of marriage. To most women, this is expensive and you have to be sure and wait for some years before embarking on it.

> The problem is that there are few marriages that have church weddings. Most families just bless their marriages after a time. And if they have just come to bless a marriage, it is a sign that they had some problems, for example promiscuity. We want to encourage youths to put emphasis on new weddings.[227]

From a few women who have had church weddings, their comment was that though they had such counselling, the church does not expand on sexuality and is not detailed. Most women commented that they do not get any sexual instructions if they miss the church weddings.[228] Probably this was why most women responded that they receive no counselling from their church on sexual and reproductive health.[229]

---

[226] *Mwina atsikana, maukwati atsopanowa. Ife sitinalandire uphungu uliwonse okhudzana ndi kugonana.* A comment from participants during group discussion at Mpira Prayer House.

[227] Int. Fr. John Mchakama, St Mary's parish priest, Chinamwali, 15.3.2005. *Vuto limene lilipo maukwati anyuwani ndi wochepa. Ambiri amangodalitsa chabe. Ngati wadzagodalitsa ndiye kuti anali ndi vuto, mwachitsanzo woyendayenda*

[228] On bedroom instructions, see Fulata Moyo, "How to be Sexually Sexy—the Church way: The Case of the Bedroom Instructions", paper presentation.

[229] Int. Women congregation from Domasi Anglican prayer house, Domasi, 18.1.2005; Mothers union members from St George parish, Zomba, 27.1.2005; Women congregation from Mpira prayer house, Mpira, 20.2.2005; Women members from Chinamwali parish, Chinamwali, 20.3.2005.

Even dogs and chicken do it without being instructed. This is the same with people. It is automatic that when a naked man sees a naked woman, *amadzuka* ([his penis] wakes up).[230]

Also, included in pre-marriage counselling is teaching on bedroom instructions, though it is often limited to ritual. On bedroom instructions, it is the duty of the officiating priest to counsel the newly wed couples on sexual life, when to make love and when to abstain sexually for instance when the woman is menstruating.[231] Mostly what is said is the passage from 1st Corinthians 7 that says that the couple should not deny each other sexual intercourse. One Anglican woman who underwent these bedroom instructions spoke as follows.

> I had my wedding in 1996. On counselling, what I was told was when you are in the bedroom, remove your clothes on your own, do not wait for the man. Not to deny the man, not to sleep with a night dress or a petticoat. I was also told that a woman needs to be keeping a pail of water in the bedroom, pieces of cloth for wiping each other and a piece of soap.[232]

The prospective couple is told to appreciate sex as a gift from God and that they need to cherish and treasure it. The clergy emphasized that not denying a man sex does not mean force but rather mutual agreement.[233] "It should not be like an office work or a job, daily. You may agree as a couple when to have sex, set a timetable, for example twice a week. Do not just do it anyhow without setting time."[234]

---

[230] Int. Agnes Mkoko, MU coordinator, Malosa, 12.1.2005.

[231] Int. Fr. Thom Mpinga, Chingwenya parish priest, Chilema, 28.1.2005.

[232] Int. NN. *Mkazi sawuzidwa chochita ku chipinda.* (A woman is not told what to do in the bedroom). *Ukafika kuchipinda kumavula wekha osadikira mwamuna. Osamukanira mwamuna, osamagona ndi night dress kapena pitikoti. Ndinawuzidwaso kuti mzimayi amayenera kumasunga ndi kandowa kamadzi ku chipinda, tinsalu topukutilana ndi kasopo.*

[233] Int. Fr. Mchakama, Chinamwali, 15.3.2005.

[234] Ibid. Despite the above comment from the priest, not even a single woman admitted to have had a timetable or at least set days for sexual activities in her home. Sexual intercourse just happens abruptly and sometimes unplanned.

Couples need to understand each other and to accept the other party's concern for example when tired and sick.[235] Both the man and the woman are advised to initiate sexual intercourse. When a woman wants sex from her husband, she is very free to ask for it. This is the same with the man.[236] Commenting on *mwambo* given to the bride only, the archdeaconry leader said that this is not right and shows that there is an anomaly somewhere. Both the groom and the bride need to be given *mwambo* together.

> 1st Corinthians 7 says we should not refuse each other for fear of Satan. On our part, we need to change. When we are wedding couples, we fail, we counsel the bride only from St Agnes. We are failing. Let us correct this. We should counsel both the groom and the bride together. Let us start.[237]

The bride is also counselled, among others, on maintenance of the new home. This includes taking care of the house, surroundings and other house chores. The care for their own bodies is also very important. The archdeaconry leader noted that some men today are divorcing their wives after losing interest in them.

> Let us bathe, ladies, taking care of our bodies that a man should not lose interest. There are some women who just get married and that is also the end of bathing. Not bothering to take care of themselves saying I have found my man. They forget that a man moves around; meeting women everyday of different sorts, some ever so smart.

---

[235] Ibid.

[236] Int. Agnes Mkoko, MU coordinator, Malosa, 12.1.2005. Cf. Rachel Nya-Gondwe Banda, *Women of Bible and Culture. Baptist Convention Women in Southern Malawi*, Zomba: Kachere, 2005. Banda found that such issues are not taught in traditional culture. My own findings reflect the same idea, that sex is the responsibility of the man and the woman should not engineer it in any way.

[237] Int. Mrs Yadidi, Archdeaconry leader, Matawale, 15.1.2005. *Pa 1 Akorinto 7 amati musakanizane kuopa satana. Kumbali yathu tiyeni tikonze. Pomanga ukwati timalakwa, timalangiza mkwatibwi yekha wa St Agnes. Tikulakwitsa. Tikonze tiziwalangiza onse pamodzi. Tiyambe.*

Let us save our marriages. A man should not slip away from our hands deliberately because of filth.[238]

The St. Agnes girls about to wed are advised that the size of the family is in the hands of the parties involved. It is up to them to discuss how many children they would want to have. However, they are not told that marriage is to bear children for fear of tomorrow if one or both are barren.[239] The girls are strongly challenged not to bring in a *fisi* (hyena) should their husband appear to be infertile.[240] Emphasis is made that marriage should not break because of lack of children, as children are just a blessing, a gift from God.[241] The newly wed family is advised that marriage is not primarily for procreation but to do what God's plan for marriage is, that is to be "helpers."[242] The clergy commented that though they do not specify the number of children in a family, the couple is advised to have a reasonable and manageable family size.

Partly yes, because you used to have free sexual relationship when they were only two of you in the house. When God has blessed you with children, you realize that it has become a bit problematic to have sex anyhow. You can't have it in the sitting room, or even during day, since the children may want to have your attention. That system of freedom goes away and you start thinking that the children are becoming a burden.[243]

---

[238] Ibid. *Azimayi tizisamba, kumadzisamala that a man asamanthe chidwi. Pali ena azimayi akangoti akwatiwa, basi kusamba kwathera pomwepo. Osadzisamaliranso ali basi nda mpata. Amayiwala kutl mwamuna amayenda, amakumana ndi azimayi tsiku lililonse osiyanasiyana ena osamba bwino. Tiyeni tisamale banja. Asatipulumuke mwamuna dala chifukwa cha uve.*

[239] Int. Ella Mhone, St Agnes coordinator, Malosa, 12.1.2005.

[240] Ibid.

[241] Ibid.

[242] Int. Fr. Thom Mpinga, Chingwenya parish priest, Chilema, 28.1.2005.

[243] Int. Fr. Brightone Malasa, Malosa, 2.3.2005.

87

Women's Sexual Reproductive Health and the Church's Pastoral Ministry

The Anglican Church is involved in a number of teachings as far as the human being is concerned. They are involved in what they call wholistic ministry, a ministry that targets the whole human being.[244] The clergy observed that they depend upon their Women Desk to deal with issues of sexuality. Members of the clergy believe not only in the distribution of labour but also that women will always feel comfortable talking to fellow women on issues pertaining to sexuality. One drawback of this is that the responsible women are sometimes busy with their office work. As a result, the employed workers may visit a parish once in a year. The clergy admitted not to have done much as a church in this area of women's sexual reproductive health. Much of what they do is to sensitize couples to be faithful to each other through preaching and marriage counselling.

> We should not cheat. There is not much we have done in that area; otherwise there are problems in most homes. And because of marriage vows, couples are forced to stick to a partner they do not like and love. Unsafe sex is common in our society and a big problem is that women do not have power to ask a man to use a condom. This is why HIV/Aids has spread so fast and is still spreading. It is like a cycle.[245]

In the Anglican Church, there are counsellors *(alangizi)* primarily dealing with marriage issues. Most of these are from the MU. In the presence of a priest, a woman cannot express herself fully about bedroom issues and in most cases, she remains silent and prefers to visit an elderly woman.[246] However, even the clergy are welcome to do marital counseling when need arises and depending on their time.[247]

---

[244] Ibid.

[245] Int. Fr. Francis Chipala, Liwonde, 28.1.2005.

[246] Int. Fr. Martin Mgeni, Mangochi, 28.7.2005.

[247] Ibid.

Family life education in the Anglican Church

Family life education is basically sex education. Following complaints from many families on marital issues, the Anglican Church in the Upper Shire Diocese decided to introduce ways of teaching couples about sexuality, with the intention of trying to make married life more enjoyable. Besides, the church noted that couples in most homes are not knowledgeable enough on sexual intercourse.[248] At the diocesan level, this type of workshop takes place once a year. In 2004, it was held in Mangochi.

> We discuss issues like how do couples interact in the home. What about communication? How do couples make the budget in the home? Aids - how does a family handle it?[249]

On the same, another priest talked as follows on one of the marriage seminars he had in his parish.

> I did a workshop once last year in my parish following marital problems presented by many women. Such issues concerned money and other marital problems. As a priest, I called all couples and we had a wonderful time. The workshop also resulted in most families that were not blessed in the church to do so. It is my desire as a priest to be exemplary in my parish.[250]

Family life education is primarily for those married. Although there are some components for youths especially those about to get married, these are tackled during St Agnes and youth conferences.[251] Anglican women commented to have heard of such workshops but expressed sentiments that only a few representatives are selected to attend. The clergy commented that because this is just a new phenomenon, only few families and mostly members of the clergy are represented. The priests further argued that this selection, however, considers different parishes and prayer houses within the diocese. The aim is that after

---

[248] Ibid.

[249] Ibid.

[250] Int. Fr. Thom Mpinga, Chingwenya parish priest, Chilema, 28.1.2005.

[251] Int. Fr. Francis Chipala, Liwonde, 28.1.2005.

coming back, they will be able to teach their fellow members in their different parishes and prayer houses.[252]

> I have been in Zimbabwe and I have seen how marriage counselling is done. Aah, wonderful. People are very united. Men and women come in large numbers. But here in Malawi, though the effort is being done, there is a low turn up. *Timachedwa tikamayamba zinthu*. We are always late when starting something.[253]

Most members of the clergy commented that there is an indication that most couples do not know much as far as sexual relations are concerned. They stated that currently they are receiving convincing remarks from the participants, that now, after the workshop, they have a satisfactory sexual life and really appreciate how good sexual intercourse is.[254] At such workshops, some of the issues raised by women include that they do not enjoy sexual intercourse because their partners are mostly too fast and seem not to know how to handle a woman in bed. One objective of this workshop is to impart sex knowledge in terms of different styles couples could use during sexual intercourse and how to arouse each other through foreplay in order to make the activity enjoyable to both partners.[255] The clergy noted that this is one way of mending marriages that seem to be on breach.

> They should try as much as possible to please each other. *Abambo apeze njira zawo, amayinso* (the men should find their methods, same with women) for example, changing styles when having sexual

---

[252] Int. Fr. Brightone Malasa, Malosa, 2.3.2005.

[253] Int. Mrs Yadidi, Archdeaconry leader, Matawale, 15.1.2005.

[254] Int. Fr. Francis Chipala, Fr. Brightone Malasa, Fr. Thom Mpinga and Fr. Martin Mgeni. Findings from the previous chapter reveal an element of failure to enjoy sexual intercourse by some women who believe their partners are not experienced and do it as if it is a fight. The priests too added that some married couples do not know much about sexual intercourse and do not enjoy it much. Nevertheless, despite this mentality, there is still positive evidence from my findings of couples enjoying sex even without marriage seminars.

[255] See appendix 4 for an example of guidelines to make sexual intercourse enjoyable. For details on foreplay, see Kristina Baker and Honor Ward, *Aids, Sex and Family Planning*, Achimota: Africa Christian Press, 1989, pp. 32-35.

intercourse. A child should not sleep in the middle. The two are one body and the baby should not be a burden to sexual life.[256]

During such trainings, men and women realize that God created man and woman differently.[257] And since they are different biologically, they also have different levels of sexual desire.[258] The clergy commented that it is their desire to reach many families with this type of workshop should funds permit.

The wife is to keep the marriage

Good behaviour is very vital to a woman in order to maintain her marriage.[259] Members of MU observed that it is the wife who keeps the marriage. To them, sometimes men leave their wives because of their behaviour as some women are always moody and bad tempered. It should be noted that this philosophy that the wife's behaviour is what

---

[256] Int. Agnes Mkoko, MU coordinator, Malosa, 12.1.2005. In relation to the *kutenga mwana* ritual, couples abstain from sex for a period of at least six to seven months before the ritual is conducted. See chapter 2. Some couples place a child in the middle of the two to act as a block against sexual intercourse before the ritual is done. The Anglican Church does not promote such a tradition.

[257] See Hilary Mijoga, "Gender Differentiation in the Bible: Created and Recognized" in *Journal of Humanities*, no. 13, UNIMA, 1999, p. 87. Reprinted in Jonathan Nkhoma, *The Significance of the Dead Sea Scrolls and other Essays. Biblical and Early Christianity Studies from Malawi*, Mzuzu: Mzuni Press, 2013, pp. 174-198.

[258] Int. Brightone Malasa, Malosa, 2.3.2005. It should be noted that this statement is from the teachers' side. It was unfortunate that I could not find any evidence from participants as very few women have participated in such training, most of them leaders.

[259] On characteristics of a real woman, see *Maria Saur, Linda Semu and Stella Hauya Ndau, Nkhanza: Listening to People's Voices, A Study of Gender-Based Violence (Nkhanza) in three Districts of Malawi, Zomba: Kachere, 2005*, p. 41. Four main categories of a real woman according to this book include, personality traits, relationship with her husband, household responsibilities, sexual attributes and fertility. On personality, the book cites, well mannered, God-fearing, trustworthy and not a gossiper.

counts is not the teaching of the Anglican Church, which believes in sexual equality and that couples are to make their marriages good. Probably, this teaching is borrowed from cultural ideology.[260]

> We are also to blame: we are moody; we are indulging in chatterbox behaviour; we remain angry up to the bedroom, depriving the man of sexual intercourse. This is not respect. Agree mutually and give yourselves timetables.[261]

The Archdeaconry leader commented that marriage is what you yourself make of as a woman. Anglican women are to set an example on respecting their marriages.

> Marriage, it is on you to keep it going. A married woman has the responsibility of taking care of the husband. If he wants sexual intercourse, *udzipeleke* (give yourself to him). Sometimes, men leave us because of lack of happiness.[262]

One Anglican woman commented that when her husband has done something wrong to her, she has the right to refuse him sex and not just to sleep with him for appeasement.

> We women are so weak. The whole afternoon being beaten, when it is dark he starts touching your body and you comply. Saying marriage is perseverance. This is not love. My husband cannot dare do that. He cannot wrong me thinking this will end in the bedroom. I cannot allow that stupidity until he kneels and confesses. Whether

---

[260] There is a danger of a woman keeping the marriage if the behaviour of one or both is unhealthy. This may reap HIV/Aids results.

[261] Int. Mrs Ndarama, MU chair, St George's parish, Zomba, 27.1.2005. *Timalakwitsa tokha azimayi, ma mood. Kulongolora, mukakwiya mpakana kuchipinda kumukanira mwamuna, umenewu siulemu. Gwirizanani, patsanani ma time-table.* Cf. Ann K. Blanc et al, *Negotiating Reproductive Outcomes in Uganda*, Kampala: Makerere University, 1996, p. 74. The author comments of a serious concern from married women who say their refusal to give their husbands sex when they demand, brings disappointment which aggravates to divorce or separation. These women commented that divorce or separation is a situation that most can ill afford due to the importance of marriage for defining women's position in society.

[262] Int. Mrs Yadidi, Archdeaconry leader, Matawale, 15.1.2005.

it will take three months, it does not matter but until he confesses, he cannot expect sex from me.[263]

MU executive stated that happiness in marriage comes in three ways. The archdeaconry leader emphasized vividly that it is not money that can make a marriage work but common sense and prayer.

Think on your own as a woman how you can keep your marriage. Money does not build marriage, it just comes. Respect is important. Your own behaviour can build a marriage. Some women are disrespectful, chatterboxes, making the man feel gloomy in his own home, wo wo wowoooo, chatter boxes. Another thing, movements. A married woman should respect herself. Do not just move around or chatting aimlessly. Make sure you're together with your husband if possible, chat with your husband. I forgot one thing, cheerless. How you receive visitors at your home can also shape a marriage. We must not differentiate between visitors, gloomy when the visitor is from the man's side and opening teeth when the visitor is from our side. Let us love our husband, let us also love his people. Sometimes, a man becomes depressed with this type of behaviour and divorces you. Let us be careful.[264]

---

[263] Int. NN. *Azimayife timapepera kwabasi. Masana onsewa ukhalire kume-nyedwa, kukada azikugwiragwira iwe ndi kumalolera. Muli banja nkupilira, chimenechi sichikondi. Wa ine ndiye amadziwa. Sangati wandilakwira nkuma-ganiza kuti zikathera kuchipinda, sindingalore zopusazo. Mpaka agwada apepesa, kaya itha miyezi itatu, palibe kathu, koma mpaka apepese ngati afuna agone nane.*

[264] Int. Mrs Yadidi, Archdeaconry leader, Matawale, 15.1.2005. Think on your own *ngati mzimayi, kuti banja ndilisunga bwanji. Chuma sichimanga banja, chimachita kubwera. Kulemekezana nkofunika. Khalidwe lako munthu lima-manga banja. Azimayi ena alibe ulemu, kulongolola. Mwamuna kukhumata pakhomo pake pomwe, ali wo wowowowowoooo, kuli kulongolora. Chinanso kuyendayenda. Mzimayi wapabanja azidzipatsa ulemu, osangokhalira kuyenda kapena kucheza kopanda phindu. Make sure you are together with your husband if possible, chat with your husband. I forgot one thing, kukwiya. Kalandilidwe ka mlendo pakhomo kamamanga banja. Alendo tisamasiyanitse kuti akabwera akuchimuna tizikwiya, akabwera akwathu kuwonetsa mano.*

Most women commented that almost all the burden of having a bad marriage is put on the wife. When there is a dispute in the home calling for *ankhoswe*, it is usually the wife that loses because she is already weak in decision making and culture too expects her to be well mannered.

HIV/Aids and the Anglican Church

The Anglican Church has a policy on HIV/Aids as a way of breaking the silence which has been there in the church.[265] The clergy commented that the silence of the church has caused a number of deaths. Because it is not possible for the church to talk about issues of HIV/Aids in the church or on the pulpit, the diocese established a department to deal with such issues.[266] The HIV/Aids committee is chaired by a lady, Mrs Chiutula.[267]

> Aids is real and the church has Aids. In August 2004 I was privileged
> to visit Lusaka, Zambia whose Cathedral was flagged with the big
> red ribbon and some words attached to it read, "The Church has

Tinkonde mwamuna wathu, tiakondenso anthu akwawo. Nthawi zina mwamuna amakhumudwa ndi khalidwe loteleri ndi kukusiya. Tiyeni tisamale.

[265] Int. Fr. Brightone Malasa, Malosa, 2.3.2005. See appendix 5 for the policy.

[266] Following a manual is something that bars the church from discussing HIV/Aids. In passing, though, especially during preaching, HIV/Aids could be mentioned. However this is seldom. I recall one of the Anglican church services I attended at Mpira prayer house on 30.1.2005 that had a hint on HIV/Aids. The theme of the message as expounded by the officiating deacon was "Jesus is the healer." With reference to HIV/Aids, Mr Gowelo assured the gathering that God is able to heal us from all our diseases including HIV/Aids. He reminded the congregation about its duty of worshiping God through prayer, abiding by his commandments and refraining from immorality. Referring to James 5:13-16 with emphasis on effective prayer, he spoke emphatically that as followers of Christ, Christians ought to follow his example and pray for the sick instead of wasting time backbiting.

[267] I wanted to speak to the chair but unfortunately failed to contact her as she was very busy and could not be reached the time I was doing my study. Nevertheless, I managed to speak to committee members most of which were priests.

94

Aids". That inscription overwhelmed me. I hoped if we had admitted it a long time ago we could have reduced the infection rate. All what the church needs today is action; we have heard and talked much about it. God forgive us.[268]

Workshops for MU are organized often where women are told about the dangers of HIV/Aids. They are also told how to avoid it, how it is contracted and how to live positively with it.[269] The coordinator cited *uzamba* (traditional birth attendance) and bathing of a corpse as examples relating to women jobs through which one could easily get infected with HIV/Aids.

> A prayerful woman is merciful and ready to assist someone who is involved in an accident on the road and is bleeding. Even wearing of gloves is a controversial issue especially when our women mix with Muslims. They would say you are not respecting the dead body. You are not respecting the religion of others.[270]

To most members of the clergy, men are responsible for the spread of HIV/Aids and for infecting their spouses. However, the clergy believe that the only way a woman could avoid HIV/Aids is to be faithful to her husband. This is however an ideal and therefore statement. From my findings, the reality on the ground is that most women expect their husbands not to be faithful. Thus, a wife's faithfulness will not help at all if the husband is not faithful to her. Subsequently, to the unmarried woman, the weapon is abstinence. Following their doctrines, the Anglican Church believes any sex outside marriage is adultery and a sin before God. As such, women that are single for whatever reasons, be

---

[268] Int. Brightone Malasa, Malosa, 2.3.2005. Compare Kenneth R. Ross, *Following Jesus and Fighting HIV/Aids,* Edinburgh: St Andrews Press, 2002, p. 40. Ross comments that in the context of the HIV/Aids epidemic, no member of the church can be un-affected as so many brothers and sisters are infected with the virus. In his words, "if one has Aids, we all have it." It is a crisis which involves the whole membership of the church. Quoting Galatians 6:2, Ross comments that we have to bear one another's burdens and fulfill the law of Christ.

[269] Int. Agnes Mkoko, MU coordinator, Malosa, 12.1.2005.

[270] Ibid.

they widows or divorcees, are strictly called to abstain from sexual intercourse. To some this period may be indefinite until they are lucky and find another suitor to marry them again.

> Contrary to the thinking of the clergy, Anglican women said it is not possible for them to avoid HIV/Aids. Accordingly, the women said if you are unmarried and faithfully abstain, you could survive. To the married, however, this is not possible, because you cannot know if at all your partner is also faithful to you.[271]

On whether the Anglican Church could save women from HIV/Aids, the MU executive refuted that saying Christianity is what you make of it as an individual. However, they commented that there is still a great advantage of belonging to a church today in this context of HIV/Aids. Members believe that if you're truly faithful and prayerful, you can survive.[272]

> The church cannot save anyone from HIV/Aids. If you are a prostitute, you are a prostitute. You may appear spiritual and prayerful but at the same time with bad behaviour, sexual relationships even in the church. Christianity is the heart; some put it on just like clothes.[273]

The clergy also observed that the church cannot save anyone from HIV/Aids. Some priests commented that it is within the same church where there are problems, adultery and fornication.[274] In their words, the Anglican women claimed that to belong to their church in the context of HIV/Aids is beneficial. Your Christian life may change the bad behaviour of your husband through prayers. Both the clergy and MU

---

[271] For details, see *Ann K. Blanc et al, Negotiating Reproductive Outcomes in Uganda, Kampala: Makerere University, 1996*, p. 88.

[272] Int. Mrs Yadidi, Archdeaconry leader, Matawale, 15.1.2005. This too is just on an ideal world. In reality, you can not survive a promiscuous husband for long despite prayers and fasting.

[273] Ibid. *Mpingo siungapulumutse munthu ku edzi. Mkazi akakhala hule ndi hule. Amatha kukhala wa uzimu ndi wopemphera koma khalidwe lili loipa. Zibwenzi ndi mtchalitchi momwe. Chikhirisitu ndi mtima, ena amavala ngati malaya.*

[274] Int. N.N.

executive believe prayers could be an answer to one's sexual desires. Besides, when you're a Christian woman, you never get moved by the pandemic and you live by hope. When you die due to HIV/Aids, you die in body only, but in spirit you live. On the judgment day, you may attain paradise despite having died of Aids, if you were a faithful woman.[275]

> We also check if the person has relatives to care for him or her. We pray for the sick. We also check the surroundings such as the condition of the home and acquirement of food stuff. We teach the relatives how to cook and care for the sick. These patients are not only those suffering from HIV/Aids but also TB and malnutrition. We also give them some drugs and counsel some on ARVs. Orphans have guardians who take care of them. We give them soap, Vaseline, blankets and ballpoints.[276]

How to uphold marriages in this time of HIV/AIDS

The Anglican Church admitted not to have done much in this area. Apart from family life workshops, they counsel the newly wed couples to be faithful to one another. The MU commented that it is in their mandate to promote the well-being of family life. Women are the most vulnerable when it comes to Sexually Transmitted Infections including HIV/Aids. Those women with unhappy marriages and promiscuous spouses are advised not to leave the man and break up the marriage. MU is not there to break one's marriage but rather to mend it.[277]

> We pray with these women and counsel them that the most important thing is prayer. It is only when things get worse that they may seek their *ankhoswe* (family counsellors).[278]

---

[275] Comment from Mpira prayer house, 20.2.2005.

[276] Ibid.

[277] Int. Ella Mhone, St Agnes coordinator, Malosa, 12.1.2005. Indeed the MU is not there to break people's marriages. "However, today in this age of HIV/AIDS, forcing someone to keep hanging on to her promiscuous marriage could lead to nothing but death."

[278] Int. Agnes Mkoko, MU coordinator, Malosa, 12.1.2005.

Anglican women are told to respect the desires of their husbands. Refusing the husband sexual intercourse could lead him to promiscuity. In the long run, even the wife could be in danger of soliciting some venereal diseases including HIV/Aids.[279] Members of the MU are also civic educated on issues of human rights. To MU, violence against women is totally unacceptable. Women are taught to be able to tell that this is violence.[280]

> Violence against women is, for example, sleeping with your wife *kowilikiza* (continuously), six times a day.[281]

The Anglican Church and HIV Testing

Members of the clergy admitted not to have done much on sensitizing their members on HIV testing. The clergy commented that this is left in the hands of the hospital personnel at St Luke's. The concerned priests stated that though they have at times mentioned it in passing, still they have not emphasized it much. The church admits that there is great need to tell women of the need for VCT before pregnancy.

> I personally have made such appeal in the church. It is essential talking of VCT today, more especially when there is hope that after being found positive, a pregnant mother may get Nevirapin.[282] Many women, especially in the rural areas, only possess basic education. It is therefore not easy for such women to understand

---

279 Ibid.

280 For details on violence, see Maria Saur, Linda Semu and Stella Hauya Ndau, *Nkhanza: Listening to People's Voices, A Study of Gender-Based Violence (Nkhanza) in three Districts of Malawi*, Zomba: Kachere, 2005, pp. 41-44. On examples of violence against women, the three authors cited among others, forced sex, men refusing to have sex with the wife and men having sex with their wives too frequently. From the group discussion, women commented that men do not give them a break except when they are menstruating. Besides, even in the late pregnancy some men demand sex until the day when she goes to deliver. To the women this was seen as violence. See p. 43. Refer also to my findings in chapter 2.

281 Int. Agnes Mkoko, MU Coordinator, Malosa, 12.1.2005.

282 *This is now common medical practice.

such issues unless someone, whom they trust, like a Priest, comes to them and civic educates them.[283]

The Church feels it is its responsibility to make sure people go for VCT and have their blood tested.[284] The MU members commented that today there is no fear of death because even if you are positive, the virus can still be controlled with ARVs. To most women, the HIV test is important because once you know your status, it is imperative to stop giving birth for your own sake. A few, however, commented that every woman cherishes a child, and as such, the best thing is to consult your doctor how you can have a child if you're HIV positive.

The Anglican Church and Antiretroviral Drugs (ARVs)

The Anglican Church in the Upper Shire diocese commends itself for the efforts made on ARVs at their hospital. St. Luke's is one of the hospitals in the country currently distributing free ARVs. The Anglican Church intends to reach out to as many people as possible so that they can benefit from the ARV scheme.

Contraception and the Anglican Church

The teaching of the church on contraception is moderate. The Anglican Church does not have any written document on the use of contraceptives. In the policy on HIV and Aids, the use of contraception is partly addressed. The church is flexible on the use of contraceptives, as it feels there is nothing wrong with using them. It would appear on the other hand that most women do complain on the side effects of some contraceptives.[285]

The sampled Anglican women denied having heard anything on contraception either from the church and the MU. However, all women are knowledgeable of contraception from friends, the radio, and more

---

[283] Int. Fr. Brightone Malasa, Malosa, 2.3.2005.

[284] For a theological argument for compulsory testing see Klaus Fiedler, "Compulsory HIV Testing. A Christian Imperative," *Religion in Malawi* no. 14, 2007, pp. 33-39.

[285] Ibid.

especially, hospital personnel. Unlike MU members from St George who stated that following a book denies them the chance to talk about contraception, MU members from Mpira said at times during their meetings, they do discuss issues of contraception including condoms on their own initiative. Some members from Mpira prayer house seemed to be in a dilemma on the issue of contraceptives. Some of those who go for modern contraceptives do have serious side effects and fail to continue with them. Besides, those who go for traditional contraceptives such as *mkuzi* (herbal string) and natural ones said these do not always work.

For example, if the husband dies, the woman is left to suffer to fend for the children. It's unlike in the past because children were born to help farming.[286]

Anglican women however said that childbirth was in God's plan. As such they cannot stop bearing children. To them, what is necessary is counselling on child spacing.[287]

Is Birth Control a Mortal Sin?

The Anglican Church believes that artificial birth control is not a mortal sin.[288] One priest commented that birth control could be regarded as a mortal sin depending on your intentions. For instance, in the Anglican Church, abortions as a way of controlling birth are indeed a sin.[289] A

---

[286] Int. Ella Mhone, St Agnes coordinator, Malosa, 12.1.2005.

[287] A comment from members of Domasi Prayer House, 18.1.2005. Kristina Baker and Honor Ward, *Aids, Sex and Family Planning*, Achimota: Africa Christian Press, 1989, p. 27 observe that a good space between one baby and the next, and a good space after marriage before the first baby is born, is part of the preparation to help give each baby the best possible start and for a healthy family. The authors believe that using scientific methods which God has provided for his people for family planning, just as one uses medicine of other kinds, is a way of trusting God.

[288] In Catholic teachings, artificial birth control including condoms is a mortal sin as stated in the encyclical *Humana Vitae* of 1965.

[289] Int. Fr. Thom Mpinga, Chilema, 28.1.2005. Helmut Thielicke comments that birth control is ethically acceptable if carried out under the claim and under the

contraceptive that aims at destroying life is indeed unacceptable.[290] Commenting on Genesis 38:8-10, the clergy stated that ejaculation outside the vagina is not a sin. *Chokolo* (wife inheritance) was part of the Levite tradition. However, in this passage, Onan son of Judah sinned because he disobeyed God to produce offspring for his brother, not because of ejaculating outside the vagina.

> Then Judah said to Onan, "Lie with your brother's wife and fulfill your duty to her as a brother-in-law to produce offspring for your brother." But Onan knew that the offspring would not be his; so, whenever he lay with his brother's wife, he spilled his semen on the ground to keep from producing offspring for his brother. What he did was wicked in the Lord's sight; so, he put him to death also (Gen 38:10 NIV).

To a few members of the clergy, birth control due to poor standards of living is a sin before God. To them, this is a sign of lack of trust in God because if there is any problem, God himself will take care of it and the children.[291] However, to most members of the church, birth control is very important but it depends on the context.[292]

> There is nothing wrong with contraceptives. However, it depends on the context. When God said go and multiply, he meant inside marriage. Child spacing is very important as it gives women time to

---

judgement of the order of creation and as one bows in responsibility to the order of creation, to the moral responsibility. See Helmut Thielicke, *The Ethics of Sex*, New York: Harper and Row, 1964 , p. 204. In common medical language, abortion is not considered a birth control method.

[290] Int. Fr. Thom Mpinga, Chilema, 28.1.2005.

[291] Int. Fr. Francis Chipala, Liwonde, 28.1.2005.

[292]Helmut Thielicke presents premarital and extramarital sexual intercourse as one of the factors making the question of birth control an issue of conflicting judgment. He states that sexuality loses its essential nature when practiced outside marriage, as it is a denial of one of the essential qualities of sexuality, namely a personal relationship designed to be permanent and the willingness to accept the office of parenthood. See Helmut Thielicke, *The Ethics of Sex*, New York: Harper and Row, 1964, p. 200.

rest and gather strength. They need to be given time to rest to enhance their reproductive health.[293]

According to the church, child spacing and stopping giving birth completely are two different things altogether. Birth control does not mean that marriage has lost its value. Children are fruits of the love between the two lovers. Whether children or no children, marriage must be there. The Anglican Church outlined the following as important reasons for birth control.

Life is becoming expensive nowadays and it is very hard to provide basic needs to a big family such as food and education.

HIV/Aids has resulted in deaths of parents leaving many children as orphans. It is a burden to those who take care of them, since they are added to the already big family they have.

There are many complications during delivery these days. This has led to many deaths.

#Lack of employment.

Lack of enough land for farming.

The Anglican Church admitted not to have done much to counsel or help widows and divorcees on contraceptives. The clergy further admitted not to have done much counselling on the use of contraceptives to women that are HIV positive. The clergy argued that the problem is that it is difficult to tell who is HIV positive.

> You will agree with me that no woman would dare share her HIV status to someone in this world of discrimination and stigma. Had it been we are in a free world and that we all accept that Aids is like any other disease, I think we, as a church, would like to help positive women to live positively. We are yet to cope up with the situation and be free to share our problems.[294]

The clergy said there is need to encourage women to go and seek advice at the nearby health centre or hospital and make a choice of their own

---

293 Int. Fr. John Mchakama, Chinamwali, 15.3.2005.

294 Int. Brightone Malasa, Bishop's chaplain, Malosa, 2.3.2005.

on the method they would like to follow. There is need to encourage them by highlighting the importance of birth control. In these days of HIV and Aids it becomes cumbersome looking after the orphans.

Women's Sexuality and Decision Making

In the Anglican sense, what makes a woman unable to make decisions about her sexuality is culture. Traditional teachings give less power to women on sexual and reproductive health. Because of culture, most women think that decision-making is the man's job. A member from Mpira prayer house commented on an incidence where her own husband castigated her in public that she likes to ask for sexual intercourse.[295] The MU executive added that fear makes women to always be passive in sexual matters. Members gave an example of a cultural practice of advising a woman not to initiate sexual intercourse for fear of being seen as a prostitute (*hule*). "We fear to say anything as he might say, woman, you have started prostitution and have seen new things."[296]

The MU executive commented that culturally women are advised that a man is the head of the family and because of this, even when she gets sick, she is forced to cook for him.[297] To the MU, this mindset of looking at the man as the head gives the woman a low status in the family. The MU executive commented that such a practice should be discouraged. It is the woman who keeps customs not the man.[298] Some of the clergy also commented that some passages from the Bible have been interpreted in a way that gives women a low place in sexual decision making in families.

[295] See chapter 2. The husband also belongs to the same church.

[296] Domasi Anglican woman's congregation, 18.1.2005. *Timaopa kunena kuti aziti mayi mwayamba uhule ndiye mwaona zina zatsopano.*

[297] Int. Mrs Yadidi, Archdeaconry leader, Matawale, 15.1.2005.

[298] Int. Agnes Mkoko, MU Coordinator, Malosa, 12.1.2005.

> When people are entering marriage, the bride is instructed to be submissive to the husband. Remember also that women are regarded as a weaker community.[299]

The clergy added that there is gender insensitivity in most families attributed to culture. The priests commented that gender balance has some consequences to children when they grow up.

> Because of our culture, we differentiate the way we bring up a girl child and a boy child. The girl is the one to cook while the boy goes out for a walk. When the girl has done something bad it is the mother that counsels her. Children need to be brought up in the same way. The same spirit you instill into boys when they are still youth, that they are bosses, they will carry it to their families when they grow up.[300]

Anglican women commented that it is now time that women became assertive and be able to discuss with their partners about sexual and reproductive health. Commenting on whether Anglican women are given any chance to take part in decision making in the church, the MU executive disclosed that very few women are invited, and that this is only occasional. Patriarchy rules, as in most cases, the clergy (all male) does the decision-making.

> Sometimes women are invited to take part in decision-making concerning issues pertaining to the church. In most cases, it is the co-worker (MU coordinator) or the President of the MU. Even myself, the archdeaconry leader, am not invited to attend such meetings. It is important to involve a lot of women to balance up the discussion. There are some issues that men on their own cannot see the need of bringing them into discussion because they are ignorant about them. Such issues like contraceptives or sexuality in

---

[299] Int. Brightone Malasa, Bishop's chaplain, Malosa, 2.3.2005. Fr. Malasa quoted Ephesians 5:21 "Submit to one another out of reverence for Christ" and 1 Peter 3:7 "Husbands, in the same way be considerate as you live with your wives, and treat them with respect as the weaker partner and as heirs with you of the gracious gift of life, so that nothing will hinder your prayers."

[300] Int. Fr. John Mchakama, Chinamwali, 15.3.2005.

general. Women should be given the room to voice it out on their own and give comments.[301]

Some Anglican women commented that at times, once issues have been discussed by the top representatives, the women are asked to give comments if they agree to a particular issue.[302] On the other hand, the clergy blamed the women themselves for not being assertive enough and stand up for their rights. The clergy commented that it is discouraging to see that women themselves do not support one another.[303]

> The problem is with you yourselves, women. We call items from the Church to be discussed at the parish level, for example. Unfortunately issues of sexuality do not come. No one seems to be interested in the matter or perhaps they do not see any need of discussing them. Yet there are problems in families, a lot. But women prefer to keep quiet and suffer silently. Mostly, it is the initiative of the priest for such issue to be discussed. Violence cannot end in families when women are just quiet.[304]

Cultural Practices and the Stand of the Anglican Church

In the context of HIV/Aids, the Anglican Church sees some cultural practices as useless. The church strongly condemns the sexual absti-nence taboos and *fisi* among others as ways of spreading HIV/Aids. Accordingly, such practices, including the ritual of *kutenga mwana*, need to be discouraged forthwith. According to the Anglican Church, the *kutenga mwana* ritual in itself is not a bad thing but the abstinence period of about six to seven months is what is condemned. Perhaps the best that can be done is to recommend the ritual to be performed after six weeks.

While we appreciate the big role women play in giving birth and certainly believe they need to rest and get more strength, the six to

---

[301] Ibid.

[302] Anglican women from Domasi prayer house, 18.1.2005.

[303] Int. Fr. Brightone Malasa, Malosa, 2.3.2005.

[304] Int. Fr. John Mchakama, Chinamwali, 15.3.2005.

seven months of sexual abstinence after delivery is just too much. What will their husbands be doing at this time? Still waiting? For sure, they will walk out and find their own ways. It is very easy for them to go into extramarital affairs that may lead to high chances of contracting the HIV virus that causes Aids.[305]

Commenting on the taboo of no sex after menopause, the priests commented that this is useless and does not make sense. Sexual desire comes with one's body. One priest said: "Menopause does not mean the end of sexual desire and it is punishing the man.[306]

The MU executive added that such practices deliberately give the man to HIV/Aids.[307] The MU executive advises their fellow women to immediately seek family planning methods six weeks after delivery and resume sexual intercourse.[308]

> There is a rule that because of HIV/Aids, we need to correct. If we stopped some practices, others should continue as long as you keep the man in your home. For example, elongation, we stopped saying that is abuse of human rights. We need to check properly. The practice of lengthening the labia should be encouraged. We do not have to throw away everything that our parents left us. The best thing is to agree with each other.[309]

The Anglican Church follows prescribed texts for teaching and usually marital issues including sexual taboos are not discussed from the pulpit.

---

[305] Int. Brightone Malasa, Bishop's chaplain, Malosa, 2.3.2005.

[306] Int. Fr. Ernest Mphaya, Matawale, 1.5.2005. Here the priests seem to assume that such taboos exist, but most women from my sample do not know anything of this taboo. Besides, the few that are aware of it do not put it into practice.

[307] Int. Mrs Yadidi, Archdeaconry leader, Matawale, 15.1.2005.

[308] Int. Agnes Mkoko, MU coordinator, Malosa, 12.1.2005.

[309] Int. Mrs Yadidi, Archdeaconry leader, Matawale, 15.1.2005. *Pali fundo yoti malinga ndi edziyi, tiyenera tikonze. Kaya miyambo ina tinasiya, awo ali ndi miyambo yawo apitilire bola asunge mwamuna m'nyumba. Kukoka, mwachitsanzo kunasiyika akuti abusing. Tiyenera tiwunike bwino bwino. Zokoka ziyenera zipitilire. Tisataye zonse anatiuza makolo, chachikulu tizigwirizana.*

Since it is also not in their pattern to visit villages, preaching against cultural practices, members of the clergy say they wait for the people themselves to approach them.[310] Usually, sexual taboos are tackled during counselling on marital problems.[311]

> People find you as a church, whether a woman or a man. Then we call them both as a family. We counsel them. This is where we give counselling services. It is difficult as a church to go to a village and talk about such issues. That is why we wait for the stories to reach us.[312]

The Anglican Church and Condom Use

The clergy commented that women with family problems such as promiscuous husbands should be strongly advised to use condoms when they are not sure of the whereabouts of their husbands.[313] Condom use should be encouraged for both the husband and the wife. The church admitted that women are more vulnerable to HIV/Aids. Because of poverty, most women find it hard to say they want safe sex. In order to safeguard the life of the innocent wife, it is important to use a condom.

> Now we have strong teams known as HIV/Aids Committee at Diocesan and Parish levels. These committees are responsible for sensitizing the general public on the importance of safe sex. I am glad to report here that of course it is hard to measure how far we

---

[310] Int. Fr Ernest Mphaya, Matawale, 1.5.2005.

[311] Ibid.

[312] Ibid. *Amakupeza anthu monga Mpingo, kaya ndi amayi, kaya ndi abambo. Ndiye timawaitana onse pamodzi monga banja. Timawalangiza. Uphungu umapelekedwera pamenepa. Zimakhala povuta monga Mpingo kupita kumudzi kukanena nkhani zimenezo. Ndiye nchifukwa chake timadikira kuti nkhanizo zichite kutipeza.*

[313] Compare Jean Garland, *Aids is Real and it's in our Church*, Bukuru: African Christian Textbooks, 2003. Garland in echo with the sentiments from the Anglican church, argues that condoms in marriage could be used when one or both of the partners are infected with HIV or one is worried that the other may be infected due to unfaithfulness outside marriage.

have gone but we are proud that we are doing something towards curbing the epidemic by highlighting safe sex as a weapon in fighting it.[314]

The stand of the Anglican Church is that condoms should be used in the marriage context when one spouse is diagnosed HIV positive and the other is not infected. Even when both are positive, they are encouraged to use condoms. It is not yet resolved to allow any other persons apart from those in wedlock to use condoms. The church strictly emphasizes that condom use is only for the married.[315] According to MU representatives, a condom is not a solution to HIV/AIDS.[316]

> . We do not emphasize condoms. The best thing is to abstain. A condom is put at the end.[317]

From the sampled women, only four have once used a condom as a contraceptive and none to prevent infection. Their reason was emergency, after they had forgotten to seek contraceptives from the hospital. One woman commented that she once sought condoms from Domasi Rural Hospital when the contraceptive she was looking for was

---

[314] Ibid.

For a different consideration see: Klaus Fiedler, "The Moralities of Condom [315] Use. Theological Considerations," *Religion in Malawi* 2006, pp. 32-37.

[316] For comparative analysis, see Jean Garland, *Aids is Real and it's in our Church*, Bukuru: African Christian Textbooks, 2003, p. 177. Garland believes promoting condoms can encourage to disobey God's law. She backs up her argument by quoting the declaration of the All Africa Church and Aids Consultation in Kampala, Uganda that said, "We believe that the prevention of Aids is best promoted in God's ideal of fidelity and faithfulness in monogamous marriage and sexual abstinence before marriage...When physical life can be preserved in the midst of consequences, we recognize that condoms may reduce risk, but we believe that promotion of condoms as the primary prevention of Aids falls short of God's ideal for the sanctity and joy of sexual fulfillment in marriage."

[317] Int. Mrs Njinga, Likwenu parish MU chairman, Mang'anda village, 12.3.2005. *Sitilimbikitsa kondomu. Chofunika ndi kudziletsa. Kondomu timaiika kumapeto*

not available on that day.[318] Women from Domasi Prayer House commented that they can influence their husbands to use condoms if need be. On the contrary those from Mpira said this is not possible.[319]

> On a battlefield, you do not choose what weapon to use. You pick anything as long as you survive. Whether it is a stone, a stick, or a *panga* knife. A condom is like a defensive weapon.[320]

The condom issue remains very controversial. One member of MU executive commented that people do still have negative attitudes about condoms.[321] The archdeaconry leader cited her own example of this negativity when she was conducting a research at St Mary's location in Zomba last year. The research that dealt with the distribution of condoms to households proved a failure because of the low response she got from her fellow women.

> I walked the whole of St Mary's, everyone refusing. Only one woman accepted them. All were saying men refuse. Some saying I am teaching women prostitution. The problem is not with men, let us not be deceived, the problem is us women. We try teaching women the benefit of using a condom, even at annual meetings, we

---

[318] This is common especially in health centres where they have specific days to seek particular contraceptives.

[319] See chapter 2.

[320] Int. Fr. Martin Mgeni, Malosa, 20.6.04. *Pankhondo sitimasankha chida chotola. Timatola chili chonse bola upulumuke. Kaya ndi mwala, kaya mtengo, chikwanje. Kondomu ili ngati chida chodzitetezera.*

[321] Compare Jean Garland, Aids is Real and it's in our Church, Bukuru: African Christian Textbooks, 2003, p. 179. She explains that people who campaign against condoms and argue that the very small HIV virus can pass through the pores (invisible holes) of the condom are weak in argument. According to Garland, though it is true that the pores in a condom are much bigger than the virus itself, HIV is very unlikely to pass through these holes as it is always attached to cells in the semen, vaginal fluid or blood. It is not floating free in the fluid and therefore is not able to pass through the condom on its own. She further comments that the cells to which the HIV virus attaches itself are bigger than the condom pores.

explain all these stories. But everyone seems not to care, just saying men refuse.[322]

The Mothers Union of the Anglican Church comprises not only those married but also divorcees and widows if they wish to join. Though condoms are strictly for those married according to the Anglican Church doctrine, talks on condoms is non-discriminatory and has no respect to one's status.

> When we are talking about the condom issue, we do not differentiate that this one is a widow or a divorcee, then she must leave the place that she should not listen to the talk. Everyone has to know. That is why we have incorporated the unmarried in the MU. Marriage is church. [323]

The Church Improving Women's Sexual Reproductive Health

The Anglican Church calendar contains a day once a year set aside to talk of creation including reproductive health. According to some priests, the challenge they have is that they do not have specific time and specialized people to focus on reproductive health as a subject. Most of the priests are lay people in the field. Thus, they depend much on their clinically trained personnel in their hospitals and health centres. In the church, this normally depends on the initiative and judgment of

---

[322] Int. Mrs Yadidi, Archdeaconry leader, Matawale, 15.1.2005. *Ndinayenda St Mary's yonse, aliyense kukana. Mzimayi mmodzi yekha ndi amene analandira. Onse kumangoti azibambo amakana. Ena ati ndikuphunzitsa azimayi uhule. Vuto si azibambo ayi. Tisawanamizire, vuto ndi ife amayi. Timayesetsa kuwaphunzitsa azimayi ubwino wogwiritsa ntchito kondomu, even at annual meetings, timafotokoza nkhani zimenezi. Koma aliyense amawoneka kuti sizimamukhudza, kumangoti azibambo amakana.*

[323] Ibid. *Tikamakamba za kondomu sitisiyanitsa kuti kaya uyu ndi wamasiye kaya osiyidwa, ndiye achoke kaye asave nawo, ayi. Ali yense ayenera kudziwa.*

the presiding priest,[324] and usually, with little knowledge on the issue, in most cases the day is not well utilized.[325]

> Girls need to be educated in the same way as boys. We do not have to differentiate the two even in the allocation of jobs—that a girl should be the one to cook while the boy goes to play football. Starting with the father, he should be able to support his wife with the house chores. If you have boys in the home, they will be able to clean pots and cook because their father does it too. You come to my home one day. You will be surprised to find me mopping the floor. When people find me, they get surprised, saying, pastor, what are you doing? Where is your wife? I know they cannot understand seeing their pastor helping his wife with the house chores, but that is a good example to my children especially the boys.[326]

> Providing alternative ways how our women can sustain their lives could be another way of improving their sexual life as they will not be fully relying on men for support. Women should support their husbands by finding ways of getting money to use at their home. They should not just wait for the man to do everything.[327] This will involve providing small-scale loans to them.[328]

> Even mipando yaikulu mtchalitchi (big positions in the church). In most cases it is men who dominate and possess the leading positions. For the first time in my parish, we have chosen a woman to be the chairperson. But that was because of my initiative; otherwise even her fellow women were ready to choose a man as the chairman.[329]

Some members of the clergy commented that there is need for inculturation and to revisit the Bible. Bearing in mind that we are living in a totally different culture, the scriptures need to be exegeted to apply

---

[324] Int. Charles Makwenda, Zomba Theological College, 16.8.2005.

[325] Int. Brightone Malasa, Malosa, 2.3.2005.

[326] Int. Fr. John Mchakama, Chinamwali, 15.3.2005.

[327] Int. Agnes Mkoko, MU coordinator, Malosa, 12.1.2005.

[328] This seems to be a good idea, but it was not indicated who should be providing the loans.

[329] Int. Agnes Mkoko, MU coordinator, Malosa, 12.1.2005.

to a particular context and time. According to some members of the clergy, it is the responsibility of the church to check its doctrines and teach appropriate messages relevant to a particular context.[330]

> The Bible is a guide in our everyday life. It was written from a different environment, understanding and purpose. We can go back to the Bible and accommodate some issues to suit a particular situation. Of course, not running away from the scripture. But an umbrella is not necessary in summer.[331]

On support given to unmarried women, the MU executive commented that singles are encouraged to be self-reliant and engage in small businesses such as farming to support themselves instead of relying on men. Nevertheless, some of the representatives commented that this is not always easy due to lack of capital to start a business.[332] The clergy admitted not to have given any support to the unmarried women. To this they added that it is necessary that something should be done to the unmarried on their sexual health, for example those that are sexually active.

> This is a big job for the church. Most unmarried are widows with children. This is why some women resort to promiscuity because they have nothing to support the children. At times, I ask myself, what we are doing as a church towards such women. All we do is backbiting, calling them prostitutes without really understanding their problem and trying to find a solution. Perhaps our support as a church is insufficient. We need to sit down as a church and reflect on the teachings of the church. Yes, our doctrines support only monogamous marriages, but how can we support the singles that are sexually active. We are now living in the time, when, quoting Bishop Aipa, "the impossible has met the possible".[333]

The clergy cited an example of economic empowerment to singles through loans as a way of supporting those that do sexual intercourse

---

[330] Int. Fr. John Mchakama, Chinamwali, 15.3.2005.

[331] Int. Fr. Francis Chipala, Liwonde, 28.1.2005.

[332] Int. Mrs Njinga, Likwenu parish MU chairman, Mang'anda village, 12.3.2005.

[333] Int. Fr. John Mchakama, Chinamwali, 15.3.2005.

for trade. The concerned priests explained that even when the church is unable to provide the loans; it has the responsibility to save its people by influencing other lending institutions to assist.[334] Commenting on the same the Bishop of the diocese spoke of a project the diocese has embarked on recently on empowering clergy wives through small scale businesses.[335] The intention is that once these wives are economically empowered they could reach out to other needy people such as widows and divorcees.

> There has been a positive response. Some have been helped. For example, at Malindi parish, the priest's wife has bought a sewing machine. We also receive donations and assistance in monetary form, money, old clothes (*kaunjika*). Our next step is to look after the singles.[336]

While some members of the clergy talked of revisiting the Bible to accommodate unmarried women, a few believe women can quench their sexual desire on their own. For instance, just as men do masturbate, unmarried women could do likewise, for example, using vibrating machines or a banana.[337] Polygamy to most members of the clergy is a channel for HIV/Aids. The Bishop, however, suggested an idea of supporting the sexuality of the unmarried by making sure that they get married.

> That is a very difficult question. No, no, no, we cannot allow promiscuity in the church. Neither can we allow polygamy. It was there in the OT but condemned in the NT. One man cannot share love. It's true, yes; sometimes we take it for granted. In Ireland, widows and widowers march on Valentine day. It is a day for the unmarried to meet. You are giving me homework. I will ask my chaplain to give me a list of unmarried women and men. For example, we can be going to our schools checking any unmarried men or widowers. Then we can arrange for a seminar for both

---

[334] Int. Fr. Francis Chipala, Liwonde, 28.1.2005.

[335] Int. His Grace Bernard Malango, Bishop of Upper Shire Diocese, Malosa, 30.3.2005.

[336] Ibid.

[337] Int. NN.

parties to meet. It's true; we have a big challenge to look after the singles in terms of their sexual desire.[338]

A few women commented that improving one's sexual and reproductive health is personal. It is up to the individual as the one who has received the word to keep it. Women need to be continuously receiving the word of God. We are different individuals and even understanding of things differs. Some grab it faster than others.[339]

Conclusion

This chapter has described how the Anglican Church interprets sexual morals in its theology. It seems there is no clear policy on issues concerning sexuality. As with culture, so in the church, issues of sexuality are taken as taboo. In most cases, pressure from outside such as marital problems forces the church to bring in the issues of sexuality. The introduction of family life education is one way of responding to family problems in most families. These workshops are meant to enlighten members on sexual life and how sexual intercourse can be pleasant and enjoyable in marriage.

---

[338] Int. His Grace Bernard Malango, Bishop of Upper Shire Diocese, Malosa, 30.3.2005.

[339] Int. Mrs Yadidi, Archdeaconry leader, Matawale, 15.1.2005.

Chapter 4: Faith versus Reality: A Diet that is not Balanced

There seems to be a gap between what the church demands and what is the reality on the ground. Messages and teachings of the church seem to be in the abstract, without achieving much on the ground. Where faith and reality are in controversy, and the diet is unbalanced, the end result is not appetizing to both sides. Culture seems to procure a big role in the society, if not outliving and bypassing the demands of the church. Culture has invaded society with its norms, beliefs and ideas and though some are not delicate, they cannot easily be erased. Thus, it is very crucial to consider culture when one exegetes the Biblical message. Rachel Fiedler comments that in the age of HIV/Aids, culture plays an important part in the way women read the New Testament. Referring to the Baptist Convention women, she notes that such women inherit messages as regards sex and marriage from their cultural point of view.[1]

Recommendations

Looking at the above scenario where faith and reality seem to clash, there is great need for enough counselling at all levels. The following recommendations to the church may perhaps help solve some of the problems. And subsequently, try to improve the sexual and reproductive life of women in this age of HIV/Aids.

Prayer for healing and daily strength should be part of our ministry to those with Aids.[2] Jesus Christ died for our sins, no matter what we have

---

[1] Rachel NyaGondwe Fiedler, Teaching the NT in the Era of HIV/Aids, paper, nd., p. 3.

[2] Jean Garland, *Aids is Real and it's in our Church*, Bukuru: *African Christian Textbooks, 2003*, p. 162. See also, Overtoun Mzunda et al, *The God of Love and Compassion: A Christian Meditation on AIDS*, Kachere, 2002. The book highlights healing of the sick and addressing the gospel message to the lost sheep to be Jesus' prime activities. Jesus wanted human beings to be healed and to be in good physical shape. Whenever we experience full health, we thankfully acknowledge God's nearness, p. 6.

done.[3] Pastoral counselling for any problem is a way of restoring those that have moved away from Christian truth and moral standards, back to what God has designed for them.[4] Praying for people living with HIV/Aids can break the silence and set a good example to the community at large for them to follow.[5] The Christian Church is always called to be a shining light in dark places, and the darker the surroundings, the brighter must the light shine.[6] Let there be a conducive environment in the church for every member including those living with HIV/Aids to have a voice and speak out their mind. It is very important that we continuously pray for love in our homes, churches, communities and in our nation. This is *agape* love.

If at all condoms could prevent HIV/Aids, there is indeed a need for the church to intervene in the condom issue. Even if condoms are not 100% effective, even if there is no such thing as safe sex, however, half a loaf

---

[3] Kristina Baker and Honor Ward, *Aids, Sex and Family Planning*, Achimota: Africa Christian Press, 1989, p. 80 comments that God can move in and make us new. He might even do the miracle of healing and save you from HIV/AIDS.

[4] Jean Garland, p. 183. The author goes on to say that a pastor who wants to shame or condemn a person, driving him away from God rather than toward God, is acting from his own sinful desire and not in a godly way. God's way of dealing with problems is to encourage us to take responsibility for our actions and situations and if necessary come to repentance and forgiveness, before moving on to healing or acceptance in that situation, p. 185.

[5] Kenneth R. Ross, *Following Jesus and Fighting HIV/Aids*, Edinburgh: St Andrew's Press, 2002, pp. 9, 10, 21. The author reminds its readers that PLWA's desire is spiritual care. Ross uses the term "Bringing words of hope under the shadow of death" (p. 21).

[6] See Kristina Baker and Honor Ward, *Aids, Sex and Family Planning*, Achimota: Africa Christian Press, 1989, p. 87. The authors comment that when a man or a woman is dying of Aids, we must not point a finger and say, "this is God's judgement" but rather remind them of God's cleansing power. They believe that, although Aids is a fatal disease, nevertheless the duration an infected person can stay alive and healthy with the virus in the blood depends on her or his personality. This could happen with enough courage and determination to live a good life, helping one's body instead of hindering it (p. 75).

of bread is better than none. May it be known to the church that sexual intercourse in our society is real, with or without a condom. Besides, let the church also consider those that are HIV positive on how they can manage their sexual life. HIV/Aids should not be a punishment to one's sexuality. They too have sexual feelings but have the sole responsibility of not spreading the virus to their sexual partners.[7] This is a big challenge to the church. It is necessary to re-examine the condoms and find out their effectiveness. Prevention is always a better and cheaper recipe than seeking a cure.

There is need for consultative meetings or seminars with men on the use of condoms. Men ought to be convinced to be using condoms. As for women, the study has found out that pressure from men and their lack of assertiveness force them not to negotiate condom use. Perhaps as the church, there is need to direct the attention to the male perspective.

Since abstinence seems to be a failure to most unmarried women (and even more men), it is very important to make sure that women are under the marriage roof where they can comfortably live their sexual lives. This is another big challenge to the church of bringing together unmarried women and men. Economic support for the unmarried through small scale businesses is also quite commendable and could at the same time pave way for self-dependence. HIV/Aids has changed the

---

[7]   On 3.7.2005 I was listening to a programme on TransWorld Radio entitled "*The Church and Hot Potatoes*" where controversial issues of the society are discussed in relation to the church. The discussion of the day was focused on HIV/Aids and Condoms. One of the pastors on the panel, condemning condom use actually posed the following question to his colleagues: "If they bring you a woman who is HIV positive and say put on a condom and sleep with her, would you do that?" I was embarrassed and felt completely betrayed. I felt ashamed in front of my family to listen to such a story. I thought it was a pathetic remark from a pastor, the same pastor who could be bridging the "gap" for me and preach a message of hope and love.

scenario of marriage, leaving widows both young and old.[8] It has also created a number of marriage break-ups.

As the church goes on with marriage seminars, faithfulness in marriage ought to be emphasized more often. From the study, most immorality is on the side of the men.[9] As such talks on the same should be conducted frequently with male members of the church.

The study also shows that both men and women do not have enough instructions on sexuality, one reason being that not many families have had church weddings where bedroom instructions, for example, are taught. Thus, those that did not have such weddings (which are the majority) are denied the relevant knowledge and instructions. It could be a good idea if the church were to disentangle sex teaching from the (usually late) church wedding, so that each person should have the chance to learn early, for example, by having pre-marriage seminars.

Finally, lack of highly nutritious food for people living with HIV/Aids has led to quite a number of deaths. Despite the government's big efforts of distributing free ARVs, they should go together with enough and right food. And for their survival, where food is scarce, even the ARVs prove a failure. This is yet another challenge to the church to make sure these patients have enough to eat.

Conclusion

As long as women are not part and parcel of decision making in the Church, issues of sexual and reproductive health will not be of prior concern to male members. Not only is women's status low in economic, cultural and social aspects, but also in their sexual and reproductive lives. Issues of sexuality are determined by cultural ideology to be the

---

[8]   In his letter to Timothy, Paul gave him, among others, instructions that young widows ought to get married in order not to be tempted by Satan (1 Timothy 5:11). The challenge is, however, when the men to marry such widows seem not to be available.

[9]   This does not rule out the fact that there are also some women that are promiscuous. However, from my study, a very small percentage of women is promiscuous so to say for reasons that could be genuine.

job of a man. Reproduction also seems to be in the hands of a man. The study reveals disparities between the morality of the church with that on the ground. This is a big challenge to the Church. It takes one's culture, religion and attitude for one to value the ABC strategy of HIV/Aids.

Bibliography

Oral Sources

Most of the interviews were anonymous. For hints on the group of women who is at the centre of this study, see appendix 1. For those interviewees who are named, see the respective footnotes.

Unpublished Sources

Bisika, Thomas et al, "Banja la Mtsogolo - Family Planning and STI Client Satisfaction Study", 2001.

Chinguwo, Evelyn, "Safe Motherhood: Constraints to Women's Utilization of Maternal Services in Zomba and Nsanje Districts", University of Malawi, 1995.

Fiedler, Rachel NyaGondwe, "Teaching the NT in the Era of HIV/Aids", unpublished.

Franklin, Funsani Hespers, "The History of T.A. Malemia, History Seminar Paper, University of Malawi, 1971/72.

Longwe, Molly, "From Chinamwali to Chilangizo: The Christianization of Pre-Christian Chewa Initiation Rites in the Baptist Convention of Malawi", MTh, University of Natal, Pietermaritzburg, 2003.

Munthali, Alister, Change and Continuity: Perceptions about Childhood Diseases among the Tumbuka of Northern Malawi, Rhodes University, 2002.

Published Sources

Abdallah, Yohana, "The Yaos: Chiikala cha Wayao," Zomba: Government Press, 1919.

Aids Epidemic Update, UNAIDS, 2004.

Ambali, Augustine, *Thirty Years in Nyasaland*, London: UMCA, 1931.

Anderson-Morshead, A.E.M., *The History of the Universities Mission to Central Africa 1859-1909*, London: UMCA, 1953

Asavaroengchai, Suwanna, "Double Standard Double Threat: HIV and Reproductive Health in Thailand" in *Private Decisions, Public Debate: Women, Reproduction and Population*, London: Panos, 1994.

Baker, Kristina and Honor Ward, *Aids, Sex and Family Planning*, Achimota: Africa Christian Press, 1989.

Banda, Rachel NyaGondwe [Fiedler], *Women of Bible and Culture. Baptist Convention Women in Southern Malawi*, Zomba: Kachere, 2005.

Berne, Eric, *Sex in Human Loving*, Harmondsworth: Penguin, 1973.

Bisika, Thomas and Paul Kakhongwe, *Research on HIV/Aids, STDs and Skin Disease in Malawi*, Zomba: Centre for Social Research, 1995.

Bisika, Thomas et el, *Banja la Mtsogolo: Family Planning and STI Client Satisfaction Study*, 2001

Blanc, Ann K. et al, *Negotiating Reproductive Outcomes in Uganda*, Kampala: Makerere University, 1996.

Blood, A.G, *The History of the Universities Mission to Central Africa*, London: UMCA, 1957.

Breugel, J.W.M. van, *Chewa Traditional Religion*, Blantyre: CLAIM-Kachere, 2001.

Central African History for the Malawi School Certificate of Education, Lilongwe: Ministry of Education and Culture, 1992.

Chakanza J.C., "The Unfinished Agenda: Puberty Rites and the Response of the Roman Catholic Church in Southern Malawi," *Religion in Malawi*, no. 5, 1995.

Chakanza J.C., *Wisdom of the People: 2000 Chinyanja Proverbs*, Blantyre: CLAIM-Kachere, 2000.

Chilowa, Wycliffe, *Demographic Projections and their Implications for Urban Housing in Malawi*, Zomba: Center for Social Research, 1996.

Chingota, Felix, "Sacraments and Sexuality", *Religion in Malawi*, no. 8, 1998.

Chipembere, Masauko, *Hero of the Nation*, ed. by Robert Rotberg, Blantyre: CLAIM-Kachere, 2000.

Chipeta, D.P. and F. Luhanga, *HIV/Aids and Health in the Teacher Education Curriculum*, Mzuzu: Olive Publishing House, 2001.

Constitution and Canons: Church of the Province of Central Africa, 1996.

Crowder, Michael, *A History of West Africa: A.D. 1000 to the Present*, London: Longman, 1979.

DeGabriele, Joseph, "When Pills Don't Work - African Illnesses, Misfortune and *Mdulo*", in *Religion in Malawi*, no 9, 1999.

Edwards, David L, *What Anglicans Believe*, Oxford: Mowbray, 1974.

Elston, Philip, "Livingstone and the Anglican Church", in Bridglal Pachai, *Livingstone. Man of Africa: Memorial Essays.*

Elston, Phillip, "A Note on the Universities' Mission to Central Africa: 1859-1914", in B. Pachai (ed), *The Early History of Malawi*, London: Longman, 1972.

Engender Health: Sexuality, Family Planning and Reproductive Health, www.engenderhealth. org/wh/sg/eswhat.html, (2004).

Fiedler, Klaus, "Compulsory HIV Testing. A Christian Imperative," *Religion in Malawi* no. 14, 2007, pp. 33-39; also in Klaus Fiedler, *Conflicted Power in Malawian Christianity: Essays Missionary and Evangelical from Malawi*, Mzuzu: Mzuni Press, 2015, pp. 35-49.

Fiedler, Klaus, "The Moralities of Condom Use. Theological Considerations," *Religion in Malawi* 2006, pp. 32-37; also in Klaus Fiedler, *Conflicted Power in Malawian Christianity: Essays Missionary and Evangelical from Malawi*, Mzuzu: Mzuni Press, 2015, pp. 22-34.

Fiedler, Klaus, "'We are all Infected or Affected' - The Moralities of Antiretroviral Treatment", *Journal of Humanities*, no. 18 (2004), pp 19-37.

Fiedler, Klaus, *Conflicted Power in Malawian Christianity: Essays Missionary and Evangelical from Malawi*, Mzuzu: Mzuni Press, 2015

Fiedler, Klaus, *Fake Healing Claims for HIV/AIDS: Traditional, Christian and Scientific*, Mzuzu: Mzuni Press, 2016.

Fiedler, Klaus, *Timange Ulalo*, Zomba: Lydia Print, 2006 (12 pp), *Let's Build the Bridge* (Lydia Print, 2006) and as *Tizenge Ulalo* [Tumbuka, 2006] and *Tuzenge Ubulalo* [Lambya, 2007];

Fiedler, Rachel NyaGondwe, *Chenjerani, Nthenda ya Edzi Ilikodi*, Zomba: Lydia Print, [2]2007; *Be Careful, AIDS is Real,* 2006.

Fiedler, Rachel NyaGondwe, *Coming of Age. A Christianized Initiation among Women in Southern* Malawi, Zomba: Kachere, 2005.

Frank, Ham, *Aids in Africa: How did it ever Happen*, Zomba: Kachere, 2004.

Garland, Jean, *Aids is Real and it's in our Church*, Bukuru: African Christian Textbooks, 2003.

Gillian Paterson, *Love in a Time of AIDS: Women, Health and the Challenge of HIV*, Geneva: WCC, 1996

Hardin, Garrett, *Birth Control*, New York: Pegasus, 1970.

Häselbarth, Hans, *Christian Ethics in the African Context*, Ibadan: Daystar, 1976.

Hubley, J., *The Aids Handbook: A Guide to the Understanding of Aids and HIV*, London: Macmillan, 1990.

Jambo, Isaac Wilson, *Face to Face with Aids*, Balaka: Montfort Media, nd.

Jeke, Claudia A.J, "Fertility Preferences and Unmet Need for Family Planning," in *Malawi: Demographic Health Survey 2000*, Zomba: National Statistical Office, 2001.

Jemott, John and Miller Suzanne, Women's Reproductive Decisions in the Context of HIV infection", in Ann O'Leary and Loretta Jemott (eds), *Women and Aids: Coping and Care*.

Joe Jenkins, *Contemporary Moral Issues*, Oxford: Heinemann, 1997.

Kadzamira, John and Wycliffe Chilowa, *The Role of Health Surveillance Assistants in the Delivery of Health Services and Immunization in Malawi*, UNIMA: Centre for Social Research.

Kamwela, Bonet, *Married and no Sex Anymore. Mbulu as a Pastoral Problem in Mzimba in Northern Malawi*, Mzuzu: Luviri Press, 2019.

Kholowa, Janet and Klaus Fiedler, *In the Beginning God Created them Equal*, Blantyre: CLAIM-Kachere, 2003, p. 10.

Kholowa, Janet and Klaus Fiedler, *Mtumwi Paulo ndi Udindo wa Amayi Mumpingo*, Blantyre: CLAIM-Kachere, 2001, p. 7.

Longwe, Molly, *Growing Up. A Chewa Girls' Initiation*, Zomba: Kachere, 2006.

M'passou, Denis, *Josiah Mtekateka: From a Priest's Dog-Boy to a Bishop*, Chilema, 1979.

Malawi Fourth National Health Plan: 1999-2004, Lilongwe: Ministry of Health, 1999.

Malawi National Reproductive Health Service Delivery Guidelines, October 2001.

Malawi: Demographic and Health Survey 2000, Zomba: National Statistical Office, 2001.

Maples, E., *Chauncy Maples: Pioneer Missionary in East and Central Africa for Nineteen Years and Bishop of Likoma, Lake Nyasa*, London: Longman, 1897.

McCulloch, Mary, *A Time to Remember: The Story of the Diocese of Nyasaland*, London: University Mission to Central Africa, 1959.

Mijoga, Hilary, "Gender Differentiation in the Bible: Created and Recognized" in *Journal of Humanities*, no. 13, UNIMA, 1999. Reprinted in Jonathan Nkhoma, *The Significance of the Dead Sea Scrolls and other Essays. Biblical and Early Christianity Studies from Malawi*, Mzuzu: Mzuni Press, 2013, pp. 174-198.

Miller, David, *Living with Aids and HIV*, London: Macmillan, 1987.

Mitchell, J.C, *The Yao Village: A Study in the Social Structure of a Malawian Tribe*, Manchester University Press, 1956.

Mlenga, Moses, *Polygamy in Northern Malawi. A Christian Perspective*, Mzuzu: Mzuni Press, 2016.

M'passou, Denis, *Josiah Mtekateka: From a Priest's Dog-Boy to a Bishop*, Chilema, 1979.

Mzunda, Overton et al, *The God of Love and Compassion: A Christian Meditation on Aids*, Zomba: Kachere, 2002.

National Aids Commission, *HIV/Aids in Malawi: 2003 Estimates and Implications*, Lilongwe: January 2004

National Aids Commission, *HIV/Syphilis Sero Prevalence in Antenatal Clinic Attendees*: Malawi Sentinel Surveillance.

National AIDS Commission, *National HIV/Aids Policy: A Call to Renewed Action*, Lilongwe: NAC, October 2003.

Newell, Jonathan, "Not War but Defence of the Oppressed? Bishop Mackenzie's Skirmishes with the Yao in 1861", in Kenneth R. Ross (ed), *Faith at the Frontiers of Knowledge*, Blantyre: CLAIM-Kachere, 1998, p. 130.

O'Leary, Ann and Jemott, Loretta (eds), *Women and Aids: Coping and Care*, New York: Plenum Press, 1996.

Paas, Steven, *Chichewa-Chinyanja English Dictionary*, Blantyre: CLAIM-Kachere, 2004.

Pachai, Bridglal, *Livingstone Man of Africa: Memorial Essays 1873-1973*, London: Longman, 1973.

Pachai, Bridglal, *Malawi: The History of the Nation*, London: Longman, 1973.

Paterson, Gillian, *Love in Time of Aids: Women Health and the Challenge of HIV/Aids*, Geneva: WCC, 1996.

Phiri, Isabel Apawo, *Women, Presbyterianism and Patriarchy: Religious Experience of Chewa Women in Central Malawi*, Blantyre: CLAIM-Kachere, 1997.

Private Decisions, Public Debate: Women Reproduction and Population, London: Panos Publications, 1994.

Ross, Andrew C., *Blantyre Mission and the Making of Modern Malawi*, Blantyre: CLAIM-Kachere, 1996.

Ross, Kenneth R., *Following Jesus and Fighting HIV/Aids,* Edinburgh: St Andrews Press, 2002.

Rotberg, Robert I (ed), *Hero of the Nation. Chipembere of Malawi: An Autobiography*, Blantyre: CLAIM-Kachere, 2001.

Saeed, Hilda, "We Can't Stop Now: Pakistan and the Politics of Reproduction" in *Private Decisions, Public Debate: Women, Reproduction and Population,* 1994.

Saidi, Emanuel, "The Aids Epidemic in Africa: Its Detrimental Impact on the Value of Human Life," *Religion in Malawi*, no 9, 1999.

Saur, Maria Saur, Linda Semu and Stella Hauya Ndau, *Nkhanza: Listening to People's Voices, A Study of Gender-Based Violence (Nkhanza) in Three Districts of Malawi*, Zomba: Kachere, 2005.

Schoffeleers, J.M., "Livingstone and the Mang'anja Chiefs", in Bridglal Pachai, *Livingstone. Man of Africa: Memorial Essays 1873-1973*, London: Longman, p. 123.

Shepperson, George, "Livingstone and the Years of Preparation 1813-1857" in Bridglal Pachai (ed), *Livingstone. Man of Africa: Memorial Essays 1873-1973*, London: Longman, 1973.

Simmons, Jack, *Livingstone and Africa*, London: English Universities Press, 1955.

Stevens, Edward, *Making Moral Decisions*, New York: Paulist Press, 1969.

Tengatenga, James, *Church, State and Society in Malawi: The Anglican Case*, Zomba: Kachere, 2006.

The Alternative Service Book 1980, Cambridge: Cambridge University Press, 1980.

The HIV/Aids Epidemic In Malawi: The Situation and the Response", UNAIDS, August 2001.

Thielicke, Helmut, *The Ethics of Sex*, New York: Harper and Row, 1964.

Tindall, P.E.N., *A History of Central Africa*, Blantyre: Dzuka, 1988.

Torjesen, Malcolm Karl, *Women at the Crossroads: A Path beyond Feminism and Traditionalism*, Downers' Grove: InterVarsity, 1982.

UNAIDS, *Aids Epidemic Update*, December 2004.

UNAIDS, *Children and HIV/Aids: UNAIDS Briefing Paper*, Geneva: UNAIDS 1999.

van Breugel, J.W.M., *Chewa Traditional Religion*, Blantyre: CLAIM-Kachere, 2001.

Weller, John, *The Priest from the Lakeside: The Story of Leonard Kamungu of Malawi and Zambia 1877-1913*, Blantyre: CLAIM, 1971.

Wilson, G.H, *The History of the Universities Mission to Central Africa*, London: UMCA, 1955.

Appendices

Appendix 1: A Case of Study of Malemia T/A

	No of children	Age at marriage	Age now	Denomi-nation	Status
1	0	25	32	Muslim	Married
2	0	19	19	RC	Married
3	2	20	67	SDA	Widow
4	6	19	38	CCAP	Married
5	2	Forgotten	35	Muslim	Married
6	4	15	67	CCAP	Widow
7	4	16	62	CCAP	Married
8	7	21	40	CCAP	Widow
9	0	16	43	Anglican	Married
10	4	17	82	Muslim	Widow
11	2	Forgotten	58	RC	Widow
12	1	20	23	Muslim	Married
13	4	16	23	Apostolic	Married
14	8	17	51	RC	Widow
15	4	19	47	RC	Widow
16	6	17	33	CCAP	Married
17	4	Forgotten	36	RC	Divorced
18	5	19	29	Muslim	Married
19	3	21	30	CCAP	Divorced
20	6	22	40	Apostolic	Married
21	5	19	38	Muslim	Married
22	2	21	27	Anglican	Married
23	2	n/a	24	Anglican	Never married
24	5	19	39	SDA	Married
25	1	23	26	Anglican	Married

	No of children	Age at marriage	Age now	Denomi-nation	Status
26	0	n/a	29	RC	Never married
27	6	22	35	Muslim	Married
28	4	16	25	Muslim	Married
29	7	17	31	CCAP	Married
30	4	20	28	SDA	Married
31	4	19	24	CCAP	Married
32	3	17	24	Anglican	Married
33	5	16	31	Muslim	Married
34	4	21	31	CCAP	Married
35	1	Forgotten	18	CCAP	Single
36	2	Forgotten	22	CCAP	Single
37	4	19	27	Muslim	Married
38	2	17	20	Muslim	Married
39	4	18	25	Muslim	Married
40	5	Forgotten	27	UPC	Married
41	3	16	23	Muslim	Married
42	2	Forgotten	27	CCAP	Single
43	3	Forgotten	28	Muslim	Divorced
44	1	Forgotten	19	CCAP	Single
45	3	Forgotten	32	SDA	Widow
46	3	Forgotten	45	RC	Widow
47	1	Forgotten	24	Anglican	Widow
48	0	n/a	33	CCAP	Never married
49	0	25	30	RC	Widow

Appendix 2: Kusikelo Songs

1 Anakubala muzibala bwino — Parents bear [children] considerately

Chaka chino mwana, chamawa mwana — This year a child, next year a child
Kulera sati choncho — Family planning is not thus
Masiku ano zinthu zadula. x2 — These days things are expensive.

2 Lulu, mwana — Lulu, child
Lulu, mwana kuchipatala — Lulu, child at the hospital

Chorus

One: Ine nkhumbira anzanga — I envy friends
All: Eyaee — E yaee
One: Ine nkhumbira azanga — I envy friends
All: Eyayee — Eyaee
One: Ine nkhumbira azanga — I envy friends
All: Eayee kuchipatala. — Eyaee at the hospital.

3 One: Mwana akulira. — A child is crying.
All: Akulira cha? — Crying what?
One: Mumve nthenda yake. — Hear the illness.
All: Nsima. — Nsima.

Chorus

One: Dziwani — Know
All: Dziwani mfolo mayi — Know woman,
kuwononga chimanga muleke. — Stop misuse of maize.

4 Watangwanika wekha — You have made yourself busy
Pamutu pali dengu — On the head, there is a basket
Kumimba kuli mwana — On the stomach, there is a child
Kumbuyo kuli mwana — On the back, there is a child
Watangwanika wekha. — You have made yourself busy.

5 Tilere, tilere, tilere — Let us plan, plan, plan
Tilere ana athuwa tilere — Plan, our children, plan
Ndichuma cha mtsogolo, tilere x2 — They are riches of the future, plan
Yambani kulera yambani x2 — Start family planning, start x2
Tsogolo la mwana wanu, yambani — The future of your child, start
Lagona pakulera, yambani. — It lies on planning, start.

Appendix 3: The Spiral of HIV Contraction[1]

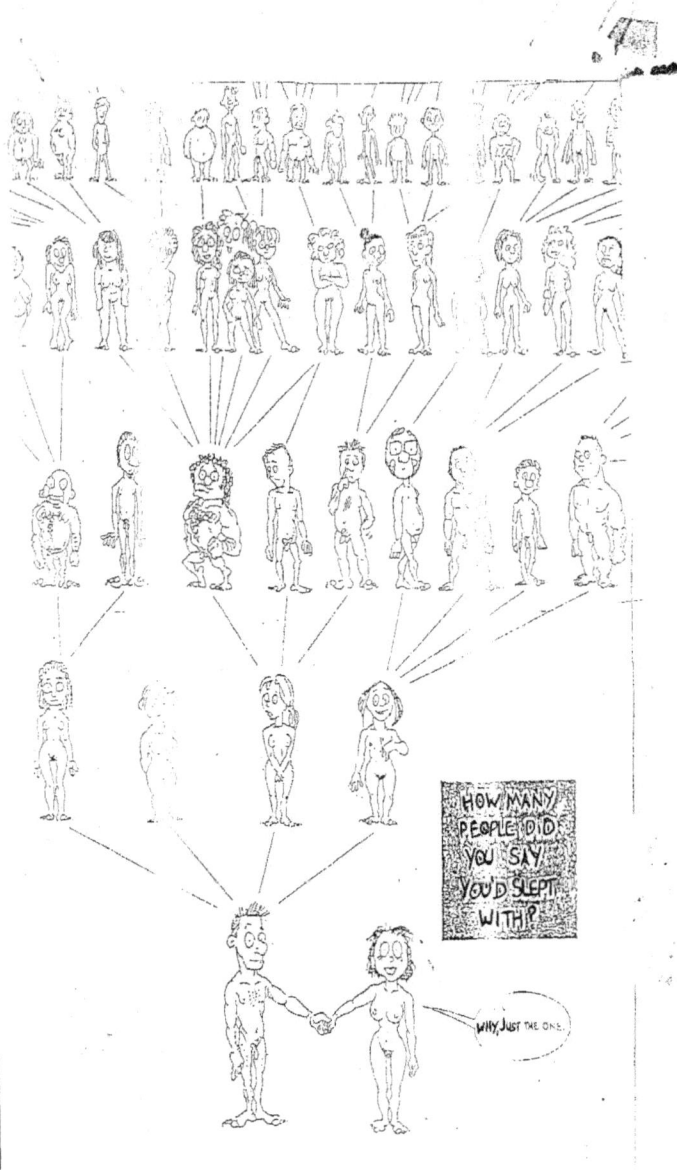

Appendix 4: Guidelines for Love Making

Mitsitsi ya Chikondi.[2]

Kodi mumatani inu bambo pogonana ndi akazi anu?

1. Ndi ntchito ya bambo kusisita mawere ndi kukoka nyini za mkazi wake kuti atenthendwe. Iyi ndi nthawi yoyamba kusisitana wina ndi mnzake. Ndi nthawinso yopatsana kisi. Mukatero mkazi amamema nyini.

2. Ndi nchito ya mkazi kuseweretsa ndi kusisita mbolo kuti mwamuna atenthedwe mokwanira. Kokani mbolo ya mwamuna wanu pang'ono pang'ono ndipo mudzaona kuti umuna ukutuluka kusonga kwa mbolo yake.

3. Ndi ntchito ya mkazi kulowetsa mbolo. Bambo adikire kufikira mkazi wake anene kuti tsopano kwerani, osangokwera ngati njinga ayi, zofunika kufatsirira bwino bwino mpaka nthawi yake ikwanire ndipo mkazi ndi amene amadziwa za nthawi.

4. Mbolo ikalowa tsopano mkazi akoke nthondo (machende) a mwamuna wake kuti akodzere bwino (kuthira umuna)

5. Sibwino bambo kuthira msanga pamene mkazi asanakwaniritsidwe. Adikire mpaka mkazi anene yekha kuti thirani.

6. Bambo ayenera kudziwa kuti pokodzerana mpamene mkazi amamva kukoma kwake kwenikweni kwa kuchindana.

7. Ndipo pokodzerana ndi pamene mkazi achepetse kunyekhulira kuti mugwirane nonse mwamphamvu kuti umuna ulowe wonse. Mkazi akapitiliza kunyekhulira ndiye kuti mwina mbolo idzuka ndipo umuna ungatayike pansi.

---

[1] Collected from Zomba VCT Centre.

[2] Written by late Rev Fr. Edgar Malunda in April 2002 in Chilema. Fr Malunda was then the Anglican Programme Director for Chilema Ecumenical Training and Conference Centre (ETCC). He died in March 2003.

8. Pamene mwakodzerana mkazi azidukulira chamkati kukhala ngati akuyamwa mbolo yabambo, koteronso bambo, kuti umuna wotsalira utheretu.

9. Ndi ntchito ya abambo kupukuta nyini ya mkazi wake ndiponso mkazi kupukuta mbolo ya mwamuna wake.

10. Mkazi awonetsetse kuti nthawi zonse pogona mbolo ya mwamuna wake ikhale m'manja kapena aipanitse muntchafu zake. Ngati mkazi wapereka mbuyo mwamuna alowetse mbolo yakumbuyo, mbolo izikhala ku nyini nthawi zonse pogona. Bambo awonetsetse kuti nthawi zonse afumbatire nyini za mkazi wake.

11. Ngati mkazi wasamba mutha kufumbatira nyini ndi mbolo. Ndipo ngati bambo atha kuyembekezera kusamba kwa mkazi wake aziseweretsa mbolo yake. Ndipo atha kuchita kisi mboloyo mochita ngati akuyamwa. Izi sizidzetsa matenda ayi. Ngakhale kuti umuna utalowa mkamwa utha kumezedwa palibe chobvuta.

12. Mukafuna kuti mukondane, kukonzekera kuziyambira patali. Muyenera kusambira limodzi, posamba kupatsana kisi, komanso kuyamwa mbolo ndi kusisitana kukonzekera kuchindana kwa madzulo.

13. Posamba bambo azisambitsa nyini za mkazi wake ndipo mkazi azisambitsa mbolo ya mwamuna wake.

Mabvuzi akakula ndi ntchito yamkazi kumeta mwamuna wake ndipo mwamuna kumeta mkazi wake. Wina asamete yekha sibwino.

The Roots of Love: What do you do when having sex with your wife?

The man should caress the breasts and pull the vagina of his wife for her to get aroused. This should be the first time for both to caress each other. It is also time to kiss each other. Once this is done, the woman offers her vagina.

The woman should play with and caress the penis of her husband to experience full arousal. Pull the penis of your husband slowly by slowly and you will see that semen comes out of the tip of the penis.

132

It is the job of the woman to put the penis in her vagina. The man must wait until the woman tells him she is ready for penetration. Do not climb the woman as if she is a bicycle. You need to be patient until is the right time, and it is the woman who knows the time.

When the penis is in deep penetration the woman should stroke the scrotum to ensure complete ejaculation.

It is not good for the man to ejaculate prematurely before the woman is satisfied. He must wait till the woman tells him to ejaculate.

The man must know that the woman enjoys sex most when the man is ejaculating.

When the man is ejaculating, the woman must reduce the rhythmic movement and they must hold each other tight so that all the semen should go. If the woman continues the rhythmic movement, then perhaps the penis comes out and the semen may be spilt on the ground.

After ejaculation, the woman should be wriggling as if sucking the penis of her husband, likewise the man, so that the remaining semen should completely go.

It is the duty of the husband to wipe and dry the vagina of his wife and of the wife to wipe the penis of the husband.

The wife must always make sure that her husband's penis is left between her thighs when sleeping [with each other]. Should she decide to offer her husband her back for sex, he should penetrate her vagina from behind. The penis must always be inside the vagina all the time when sleeping with each other. The man must make sure to clasp his wife's vagina.

If the woman is in her menses, you can touch the vagina with the penis. If the husband can wait till his wife finishes her menses, the wife should be playing with her husband's penis. And she can also kiss the penis as if sucking. This does not bring any illness. Even if semen should enter the mouth and be swallowed, there is no problem.

When you want to make love, preparation should start well in advance. The couple should take a bath together and kiss as well as caress each other in preparation for the sex that would take place in the evening.

When bathing, the husband must wash his wife's vagina while the wife must wash her husband's penis.

When the pubic hair is grown, the wife should shave her husband's and the husband his wife's. No one should do this on his or her own. It is not good.

Appendix 5: Policy Statement on HIV/Aids for the Diocese of Upper Shire

Recognizing with great concern the effect of HIV/Aids on our people, where approximately one third of the vulnerable population are infected with the virus; where the number of infections is rising rapidly, especially among young people; where the Aids pandemic is affecting all sectors of society, including the Church, and threatening progress in development, education and health care,

We, the Anglican diocese of Upper Shire commit ourselves to seriously take part in the fight against Aids. We confess that in the past, we have failed to speak out openly, we have sometimes been judgmental and unloving towards those living with Aids, and we have failed to promote vigorously the Christian values in regard to sexuality and marriage needed to protect the vulnerable against Aids.

To break the silence and remove the stigma of HIV/AIDS, recognizing that Aids is a disease and not a sin, which affects ordinary people living ordinary lives. We need to motivate our Christian congregations to speak the truth and be open about aids, and to have positive attitudes towards those living with this disease.

To promote the values of faithfulness in marriage, a healthy Christian approach to sexuality as a gift from God, and to promote behaviour change in young people, especially abstinence before marriage.

To provide care and support to those living with Aids through support groups, hoe-based care and pastoral counselling, and encouraging those living with Aids to participate fully in the life of the Church and in Aids education and care programmes.

To provide care and support to orphans, through home-based programmes, supporting guardians, and to assist widows and widowers with pastoral care and other support, and through income generating activities.

To give pre-marriage preparation and counselling, promoting pre-marriage testing, where appropriate, and relevant advice.

To provide support and help to the vulnerable, especially women and young girls, empowering them to refuse unwanted sex, trough education and support groups and economic empowerment.

To influence cultural practices which contribute to the spread of aids and ST is (Sexually transmitted infections) by enlisting the helps of community leaders and traditional practitioners, and those involved in initiation of the young.

We do not think it is the role of the Church to promote the use of condoms, especially where it undermines the message of faithfulness in marriage and pre-marital abstinence. However, we recognize that there is a role for condoms to protect the spread of this disease, and information on condom use should be made available within the context of pastoral counselling, especially within marriage where one or both partners are HIV positive. While we do not condone risk behaviour which leads to the spread of Aids, we recognize the government's responsibility in promoting condom use for those at risk in the affirmation that God loves even and especially the sinners, and anything that reduces death and suffering must conform to God's will.

Finally, we will teach and preach the love of Christ for all people and be bearers of hope and comfort to those in pain or despair, recognizing that God's love is stronger than death and nothing, not even death, can separate us from his love in Christ Jesus our Lord (Romans 8 38-39).

To carry out the above policy the diocese has established an Aids Advisory Committee and appointed a diocesan Aids co-ordinate to support parishes, Church schools and other institutions in their fight against Aids. A budget for this has been provided by USPG.

Index

Abstinence 9, 34f, 53, 57, 67f, 71f, 96, 107, 110, 119

AIDS 7-9, 17, 22f, 27, 32-34, 37-40, 42f, 51-58, 65, 67f, 72, 78f, 89-91, 93, 95-101, 103f, 107-110, 115, 117-121

Anglican Church 8, 11f, 15, 17, 47, 56, 78, 82, 85, 89f, 92f, 95-100, 102-104, 107-109, 111f, 115

Antenatal 8, 21, 27, 36, 56, 58

Antiretroviral Drugs 100

Birth experiences 35

Caesarian section 24-26

Child spacing 101, 103

Clergy 50, 54, 83-86, 88-92, 95-99, 102, 104-106, 108f, 113-115

Compassion 7, 117

Condoms 9, 33, 35-42, 52, 56f, 61f, 89, 101f, 109-111, 118f

Contraceptives 29, 34-36, 38f, 50, 100f, 103f, 106, 110

Counselling 19, 21, 85f, 89, 91, 101, 104, 108, 117f

Diet 117

Diocese 8, 14-16, 82, 84, 90, 114f

Discrimination 36, 104

Family Planning 8, 34-39, 71, 79, 91, 101, 108, 118

Forgiveness 118

HIV 7-9, 17, 22-25, 27, 32-34, 37, 39-43, 51-62, 65-68, 72, 78, 89, 93, 95-100, 103f, 107-110, 115, 117-121

HIV infection 8, 56

HIV testing 99

Hope 17, 55, 98f, 118f

Marriage counsellors 48, 69, 74, 89, 99

Mother to child transmission 9

Mothers Union 85, 111

Orphans 30, 98, 103f

Polygamy 30f, 82f, 115

Poverty 30, 109

Prayer 47, 57, 80, 85, 90f, 94f, 98f, 101, 104, 106, 110, 117

Pregnancy 18, 67

Sexual intercourse 30, 35, 37-39, 42f, 46-48, 67f, 72f, 75, 84, 86f, 90-93, 97, 99, 103f, 108, 114, 116, 119

Sexual reproductive health 7-9, 27, 52, 61, 89

Sexuality 7f, 62, 78, 81, 83, 85, 89f, 103f, 106, 115, 119f

Shame 9, 45, 73, 118

Still birth deliverie 26

Tuberculosis 59-61, 98

Virus 7, 9, 22, 40, 42, 53-61, 78, 96, 100, 107, 110f, 118f

Widow 9, 17, 30, 32-34, 44, 50, 59, 61f, 65, 97, 104, 111, 114f, 120

Witchcraft 28, 56